The Doctrine of Signatures

SCOTT BUCHANAN

THE DOCTRINE
OF SIGNATURES

A DEFENSE OF THEORY IN MEDICINE
Second Edition

Edited by Peter P. Mayock, Jr.
With a Foreword by Edmund D. Pellegrino

UNIVERSITY OF ILLINOIS PRESS
Urbana and Chicago

Introduction and Foreword © 1991 by the Board of Trustees
of the University of Illinois
Originally published in 1938 simultaneously in the United States
by Harcourt Brace and Company and in the United Kingdom
by Kegan Paul, Trench, Trubner, and Co., Ltd.

Manufactured in the United States of America
1   2   3   4   5   C   P   5   4   3   2   1

This book is printed on acid-free paper.

Library of Congress Cataloging-in-Publication Data

Buchanan, Scott Milross, 1895–1968.
    The doctrine of signatures : a defense of theory in medicine / Scott
Buchanan ; edited by Peter P. Mayock, Jr. ; with a foreword by Edward
D. Pellegrino.—2nd ed.
        p.   cm.
    Includes bibliographical references.
    Includes index.
    ISBN 0-252-01782-X (cl : alk. paper).—ISBN 0-252-06150-0 (pb : alk.
paper)
    1. Medicine—Philosophy. 2. Signatures (Medicine) I. Mayock, Peter
P., d. 1990. II. Title.
    [DNLM: 1. Philosophy, Medical. W 61 B918d]
R723.B75   1991
610'.1—dc20
DNLM/DLC
for Library of Congress   90-11127
                                                              CIP

What a piece of work is a man! how noble in reason! how infinite in faculty, in form and moving! how express and admirable in action! how like an angel in apprehension! how like a god! the beauty of the world! the paragon of animals! And yet, to me, what is this quintessence of dust?

HAMLET.

CONTENTS

FOREWORD

Prescient books often go unheralded and seem destined to obscurity. Some few germinate slowly and flourish in a later time when the intellectual climate is more propitious. Such a book is Scott Buchanan's *Doctrine of Signatures,* which has been reprinted a half century after its first publication.

In 1938 the times were uncongenial for so rarefied an effort as a general theory of medicine. The Western world was preparing for another bloody conflict. Philosophy had taken a decidedly antispeculative turn. The philosophy of medicine was a nonexistent enterprise. Buchanan's effort could hardly have surfaced in a less hospitable environment.

In the last twenty years the ground has become fertile for the germinating seed Buchanan had planted. The challenges of biomedical ethics have attracted philosophers to the more fundamental questions of the nature of medicine. The incompleteness of an ethic divorced from a theory of medicine is becoming apparent. The liberal arts are reexamining their place in the education of professionals. We are beginning to appreciate that we need what Buchanan had offered us.

While some may argue that it is a branch of the philosophy of science, the philosophy of medicine is now a legitimate area of scholarly inquiry. The logic, epistemology, and metaphysics of medicine, as well as its phenomenology and hermeneutics, now attract formal philosophical reflection. The philosophy of medicine, while still a nascent discipline, already has its own journals, a growing literature, and a dedicated coterie of scholars. In this new climate, Buchanan's book can become the powerful catalyst it could not have been in 1938.

The Doctrine of Signatures—despite its Aristotelian and Galenic orientation—is of more than antiquarian interest. It deserves the thoughtful reading of any scholar serious about developing a theory of medicine. It is still one of the very few philosophies of medicine. Many of the problems now subsumed under the rubric of the philosophy of medicine are better classified as philosophy in medicine. They are creditable studies, to be sure, but they concentrate on philosophical problems that may be particularly well exemplified in medicine but are not peculiar to it. In this category are such important and popular topics as mind-body relationships, causality, taxonomy, nosology, decision theory, decision in the face of uncertainty, theories of explanation, the epistemology of stochastic and statistical data, and risk assessment. A philosophy of medicine, properly speaking, would focus on philosophical problems peculiar to medicine as a human activity—the nature of the healing relationship; the concepts of health, disease, illness, suffering, death, and dying; the relationship of medical knowledge to knowledge in the sciences, social sciences, and humanities; the phenomena peculiar to clinical judgment; the definition of a patient's good; and the nature of trust and hope in the phenomenology of illness. It is out of these considerations that a general theory of medicine will eventually emerge, and it is in this direction Buchanan's book turns us.

Buchanan certainly did not pursue the whole agenda of topics that constitutes the philosophy of medicine today. He did, however, take up parts of that agenda imaginatively and rigorously. We may not accept his theory of signs and symptoms, which is so closely tied to the medical philosophy of Galen, but his quest for a theory of medical activity has never been more pertinent than it is today. Many of the crucial questions in the ethics, sociology, and politics of medicine are in a confused state for want of a philosophy of medicine. What we think medicine is, how we interpret the healing relationship, what we think of medicine's relationship to society and culture, and what kind of knowledge medical knowledge is are all implicit assumptions upon which far-reaching decisions and policies are being built. We cannot give rational shape to some of the most urgent questions that face us without a better idea of what it is to be a physician, what should be the ends and purposes of medicine, and what distinguishes medicine from other forms of human activity.

Buchanan did not directly address these questions. But in proposing that there could be a "strictly medical science" he set out the possibility of a theory of medicine peculiar to medicine, very much as others had set out theories of law, religion, history, or education. Despite his unapologetic Aristotelian and metaphysical stance, Buchanan anticipated some of the topics of increasing interest to philosophers of medicine today. His theory of the meaning and interpretation of signs and symbols prefigured the interest in medical semiotics and hermeneutics. His idea of the "body as artist" opened up the rich vein of thought about the phenomenon of embodiment and its ramifications in physical and emotional health and disease. His astute analysis of the essentiality of the liberal arts to the arts of the clinician is as clear an expression of the relevance of the liberal arts to the daily work of the doctor as has been advanced anywhere. Buchanan recognized that medicine is solely neither science nor art, but an amalgam of both. His proposal of the liberal arts as the bridge between the sciences and the humanities is worthy of the most serious attention by today's educators. Because of this, it is clear that the liberal arts are not mere educational adornments, but tools essential to the competent performance of the doctor's basic tasks of interpretation and reasoning from clinical signs and symptoms.

Like any truly seminal work, *The Doctrine of Signatures* will provoke, encourage, and stimulate philosophers and physicians to examine the whole medical enterprise critically. Buchanan's observations carry a particular conviction because they are based on an intimate examination of the realities of medicine and a year on the yards and the anatomy laboratories of the Johns Hopkins Medical School and Hospital. They are a model of how the philosopher can start with the realities of medicine and move to the most fundamental considerations—not as an esoteric speculative exercise but as a reflection on actual experience. Philosophers of medicine would do well to study Buchanan's method, if only to increase their ability to communicate with those in the profession they are seeking to influence.

We are indebted to Dr. Peter Maycock for his introduction and the University of Illinois Press for its reissue of this book. Its influence, one hopes, will enrich the nascent but essential efforts to evolve a philosophy of medicine congruent with the society and culture of our times.

                                        Edmund D. Pellegrino

INTRODUCTION TO THE SECOND EDITION

PETER P. MAYOCK, JR.

For over fifteen hundred years Galen's treatises were the theoretic foundation for practice by the medical profession. Though Galen was considered a mentor and practically divine, over the past three centuries his teachings have gradually vanished from schools of medicine. In 1938, *The Doctrine of Signatures* emerged to fill that void and remedy that neglect in medical theory and education.

Today's increasing health care costs and criticisms of medical education have given rise to fresh occasions for review of Buchanan's presentation of Galenic theory. He recognized that the root of these problems, then and now, is the absence of any accepted philosophy or theory of medicine. In 1981 a noted advocate for the humanistic tradition in medicine, Edmund Pellegrino, maintained that *The Doctrine of Signatures* is "one of the first and most significant works in our time that can properly be considered a formal philosophy of medicine . . . [and] a profound analysis of the nature of medicine and the thought processes crucial to its endeavors. [Buchanan's thoughts] should be pondered by every medical educator."[1] In 1987 philosopher-educator Mortimer Adler extolled the work as "an extraordinarily original contribution to the study of medicine."[2]

During the twentieth century the medical profession in the United States has been confronted by increasingly critical issues that threaten its unity and integrity. Throughout *The Doctrine of Signatures* Buchanan asked an endangered profession if society wanted courteous, rational "free-doctors" or tyrannical, empiric "slave-doctors" as characterized by Plato in his dialogue on *Laws*.[3] Externally, the medical community is besieged by socio-economic forces. Diversion of its income to administrators, insurers, government agencies, and others has weakened a major source of its independence. The ancient bond of direct fee-for-service payment between doctors and patients is disappearing rapidly. Internally, recent educational reforms have undermined training in the medical arts and sciences with a change from their firm foundations in the natural sciences to the slippery slopes of the social sciences.

Amidst these concerns about medical economics and the education of doctors there is both a social contract and a core curriculum that evades definition by practitioners, researchers, and academics in medicine. Recently, the author of *Philosophy and Medicine* reflected on the profession's naïveté: "Doctors in the main believe that they carry on their practice without employing any general theory or philosophy, either in an overt or implicit way."[4] A vague, amorphous, or unacknowledged theory of disease and a vaporous philosophy of medicine prevail to the detriment of the public, the profession, and their interrelations. Fundamental, unifying concepts seem to elude both teachers and students of modern medicine. In a 1986 issue of *Daedalus* Eric Cassell reported that medicine's theory is in transition, therefore, doctors are losing the public's confidence. He further observed, "How well a theory that is fundamental to medicine works has a profound effect on how doctors behave, on relations within the profession, on relationships with patients, and even on the power of the profession in general."[5] Furthermore, Cassell fully endorsed the conclusion of a modern historian of medicine that "professional coherence is engendered by doctrinal coherence."[6] In 1982, Thure von Uexküll, physician and heir to a tradition in semiotic, predicted that medicine's theory is currently at a dead end that can be escaped only with the help of signs.[7] *The Doctrine of Signatures* provides pathways to a restoration of sound theoretic foundations for the practice of modern medicine.

The current crisis in medicine is reminiscent of events between 1927 and 1938. American medicine during the 1920s was gaining worldwide acclaim through its achievements in many areas: the pioneering neurosurgical procedures of Harvey Cushing, multispecialty group practices exemplified by the Mayo Clinic, advances made in international health through the auspices of the Rockefeller Institute, and our first Nobel prize in medicine. But in the early thirties, because of severe, widespread unemployment and low productivity, the introduction of socialized medicine modeled on the European system seemed imminent. Indeed, in 1929 the physician-historian at the Surgeon General's Office, Fielding Garrison, had observed, "As we enter the machine age, the salient fact about medicine is the trend towards *socialization.*"[8]

Then as now, most American doctors regard the introduction of any form of government-controlled medicine as an unmitigated disaster because of its menace to their professional freedom. In a system of medicine subsidized by any third-party agency, the doctor-patient relationship would be disrupted and, in a federalized system, doctors would be relegated to the role of civil servants. As government employees, they would be subject to the whims and wishes of the political forces in power. Antithetically, many citizens look to socialized medicine as an opportunity to institutionalize their perceived right to regular and emergency medical attention. Further, within such a sociopolitical scheme, they envision that the cost of a lifetime of medical care would be borne by the community at large. Clearly,

hopes engendered by the collective notions of society conflict with the independence and traditions of an ancient profession. The signs of the times indicated that the burgeon-
ing successes of American medicine were nearing a perilous
crossroads where the dire social needs brought on by the
Great Depression would have to be resolved. Fortunately,
leaders from medicine, business, and government had already commissioned an advisory body to examine such
issues.

In May 1927, coincident with the annual meeting of the
American Medical Association, the Committee on the Cost
of Medical Care was created to institute health services research. Experts in public health under the supervision of a
Chicago-based economist published twenty-seven privately
funded reports at a cost of about $1 million. On October
21, 1932, after five years of intensive investigations, the
majority recommended that "the cost of medical care should
be placed on a group payment basis, through the use of insurance, through the use of taxation, or through the use of
both of these methods."[9] The specter of compulsory health
insurance, or "socialized medicine," incited Morris Fishbein, noted speaker for the American Medical Association,
to respond in a December 1932 editorial: "The alignment is
clear—on one side the forces representing the great foundations, public health officals and social theory—inciting to
revolution; on the other side, the organized medical profession of this country urging an orderly evaluation guided by
controlled experimentation which will observe principles
that have been found through the centuries to be necessary
to the sound practice of medicine."[10] Thus, the battle lines
were drawn between the proponents of theoretic solutions
and the advocates of pragmatic experimentation.

Shock waves from the resounding clash in Chicago were
distinctly felt by John Dewey, Ludwig Kast, and other members of the board of the Josiah Macy, Jr., Foundation in
New York, an organization devoted solely to medical re-

search and education that had partially underwritten the committee's report. Kast, then president of the foundation, found that consequences of a world war and the Great Depression indeed threatened the advent of socialized medicine. Further, he noted that medical school reforms accelerated by the Flexner reports of 1910–12 led to narrow specialization and horrid depersonalization in the practice of medicine. Kast foresaw that the developing struggle between social theorists and practicing physicians about financing the nation's health care system soon would involve principles affecting the training of doctors. So it happened that this political and economic debate sparked the initial impetus to formulate a philosophy of medicine that might reconcile societal demands without sacrificing professional integrity.

A most powerful incentive for philosophic review was provided by the untoward consequences of Flexner's detailed critiques of medical education. Based on the existing leadership and pre-eminence of German medicine, his recommendations accelerated changes throughout America's medical colleges. Laboratory and experimental sciences were given precedence over the clinical arts in schools where medicine's heritage of preceptorial and didactic teaching had traditionally prospered. Furthermore, a millennium and more of Galenic medicine had been stigmatized by Flexner as dogmatic, even infamously "scholastic" and a new era of "scientific medicine" was welcomed. An epoch of medical enlightenment seemed to have been born and was soon in full flower, as illustrated by the new school at Johns Hopkins Hospital in Baltimore, which had served since its founding in 1889 as a model to the successes attendant upon this revolution in medical theory and education. In the view of some educators, however, the next generation of doctors—products of the Flexner reforms—seemed ill-equipped to respond to the urgent social questions of the times. The draconian infusion of laboratory sciences at the expense of the clinical arts had taken its toll.

In reaction to the possible effect of some form of socialized medicine on medical education, Kast envisaged a need to strengthen students intellectually and morally so that they might take on formidable new obligations. He believed that the advocates of sociopolitical revolution had persuasive, well-developed theories on which to base reform, whereas the medical profession had little conviction and no doctrine and thus remained defenseless against the storms of societal change.

Fortuitously, Scott Buchanan, then professor of philosophy at the University of Virginia, had been engaged to give two lectures on medicine for the series "The Nature of Higher Education" at the School of the People's Institute of Cooper Union in New York City. The series included his "good companions in the larger speculative enterprise," Mortimer Adler speaking on law and Richard McKeon on theology. On January 3, 1933, Buchanan delivered his first lecture, "Medicine and the Arts and Sciences," followed five days later by "Medicine: A Philosophy of Nature." Themes developed in the institute lectures stimulated Kast's interest in this philosopher's ideas about medical education. Consequently, he initiated a dialogue on a theory of medicine that might fortify the profession in the impending engagement between the proponents of socialized medicine and the defenders of traditional modes of practice.

Kast and the directors of the Macy Foundation identified three major focuses of trouble and confusion for the profession. Primarily, they were concerned about resolving disparities between the ancient arts of medicine embodied by its practitioners and the modern sciences of medicine then being expanded exponentially by the research and academic communities. They were also alarmed at the growing gap in understanding between lay and professional personnel about medical affairs affecting the public domain. Finally, publication in 1929 of A. N. Whitehead's Gifford Lectures on "the philosophy of the organism"—*Process and Reality*—

raised disturbing questions about organic unities in humans and nature, especially for the adherents of John Dewey's ideas on nature and experiment. Kast foresaw that the breadth and depth of these problems necessitated a philosophic review.

With this background, Buchanan submitted his response in a memorandum proposing a critical investigation of the internal state of the medical arts and sciences. He intended to survey "the architecture of ideas," seeking to distinguish between arts and sciences while always preserving their unity or, as he stated in the 1938 introduction, "The power of speculation depends on a unity that comprehends diversity." In *The Doctrine of Signatures,* he conceived of this unity as arising from the analogous reasoning employed by the liberal artist and by the physician as clinical artist. In his view, the methods and operations of modern sciences—usually referred to as observation, prediction, and verification—have historically derived from the laboratory arts and sciences of the Galenic tradition—diagnosis, prognosis, and therapy. Furthermore, both professional pursuits, in the laboratory and at the bedside, reflected universal thought processes that have been refined through the ages by the philosopher and liberal artist in their works on grammar, rhetoric, and logic, later distilled into the medieval *trivium.* Buchanan perceived that a "unified organism cannot be understood without a unified intellect," thus, to accomplish the unification between the medical arts and its sciences, he appealed to Kast and the foundation for a restoration of liberal arts studies in the preprofessional and professional curriculum.

Second, in respect to lay and professional communications, Buchanan's memorandum referred to "the immensely fruitful doctrine of signatures" that claims inherent connections between symptoms and therapy. He asserted that this doctrine, nature's signatures, clarifies the complex patient-doctor interactions. His previous experience at the

People's Institute prepared the way for opening an inter-
disciplinary avenue through semiotic (though neither this
word nor *semiology* is a part of Buchanan's lexicon). During
those years he had lamented the absence of dialogue between humanists and scientists who lectured there. To
help resolve this cultural gap, he published *Poetry and
Mathematics* in 1929, which evoked analogies bridging the
universe of mathematical symbols and that of literature's
signs, in effect translating the arcane language of the *quadrivium*—arithmetic, geometry, music, and astronomy—into
the ordinary terms of the *trivium*. In *The Doctrine of Signatures,* he fashioned a semiotic by differentiating modes of
signification or levels of discourse—grammar, rhetoric, and
logic. By distinguishing first and second impositions from
first and second intentions of terms, Buchanan was able to
erect a dynamic, interpenetrative scheme of intellectual processes that order physical, mathematical, and metaphysical
concepts into a coherent system of knowledge. At this
time, he simply advised Kast that the near-forgotten, long-
neglected doctrine of signatures provided a methodology for
transforming the abtruse, technical diction of modern science and research into everyday language. Thereby he expected to close the fissure between levels of professional
and public education.

After promising to relieve the tensions between artists
and scientists and between lay and professional educators
through exercise of the liberal arts, Buchanan turned to the
third and more profound issue Kast had raised—"the organism as a whole." Not an advocate for the simpler tenets
of "holistic" medicine, he envisioned three steps in the inte-
grating process: correlation of the arts and sciences, analysis of fundamental concepts, and rational interpretation of
the data. Buchanan argued that to renew "the architecture
of ideas," which made possible modern empirical medicine
in the first place, such an alternative mode of integrative
analysis was necessary for the creation of a genuine, ra-

tional science of the human organism. At the time of the memorandum, he had not formulated other basic insights on form and matter and on teleology and final causes, which constitute a vital core of his doctrine. However, he did foresee the large and intensive effort these procedures would entail and counseled Kast on the formation of a permanent board to accomplish this "essential medico-philosophical task."

Then Buchanan explained how the genesis for his defense of medical theory arose from the ancient doctrine of signatures. Although Hippocrates is considered "the father and master of semiotic," his successor, Galen, advanced those early observational techniques to include animal and other experimentations, moving from clinic to laboratory and back.[11] Galen was resolute in his confidence of an underlying design throughout nature to be demonstrable in accord with a doctrine of signatures. This primitive mythology avowed that humanity has not been left without help for its ills; it has been supplied with appropriate remedies for disease that only need to be discovered to use nature's healing power. Further, things of nature are signed in a way that allows a trained interpreter to know that this mineral or that plant is useful or specific for this or that disease. By expanding this doctrine "rhetorically," Buchanan stated that the clinical artist is capable of reading the signs emitted by the book of nature, including human nature, and to interpret logically any necessary correctives; and just as symptoms and signs properly read by the clinical artist direct appropriate treatment for the body, so the signs and symbols of the intellect properly understood by the liberal artist lead to remedies for the soul—in this case, the soul of medicine.

Buchanan concluded his memorandum to Kast and the Macy Foundation with eleven specific prescriptions for the medical profession. Eight from this 1933 memorandum were duplicated to comprise the final declarations of *The Doctrine of Signatures.* Only one of his proposals for medical reform was absent from the 1938 printing: "A review and reinterpretation of professional and preparatory medical education in the light of the foregoing." This significant omission presaged a new responsibility in his career as educator and liberal artist.

By that time, Buchanan found that in outlining a philosophy of medicine he had at the same time laid out a blueprint for a philosophy of education. Indeed, he later commented that *The Doctrine of Signatures* required a radical reeducation for the reader. Meanwhile, he developed a curriculum of undergraduate studies that was established in 1937 as the New Program at St. John's College, Maryland. There as dean, he hoped to demonstrate that the practice of the liberal arts, exemplified by the greatest authors from Homer to Einstein, gives life to the possibilities inherent in poetry and mathematics, our most exalted means of communication. By acquiring the arts and sciences of the *trivium*, this medicine of the soul, students were to be initiated into "the Civilization of the Dialogue," a program of self-realization.

As a historical document, *The Doctrine of Signatures* reacted to two recurrent issues for medicine—economics and education. The spark that ignited its flaming light was the 1932 report on medical economics. Buchanan's response to this challenge is foreshadowed in the epigraph of this work, "what is this quintessence of dust?" and is epitomized in his final exhortation to study humanity. As he had learned from Plato that social action reflected humanity "writ large," so Buchanan concluded that resolution of social problems must be found in humanity, which is "society writ small." To him, medicine was "a universal science, humanistic in its practical aims," and he would include in his study of humanity "more troublesome branches of medical science"—"geographic medicine, industrial medicine, and even legal and religious medicine." Thereby, the profession would acknowledge that the arts of life have their natural, social, and cultural dimensions; indeed "the family physician has always had to face a total situation and the profession as a whole may well have to follow that example." His seventh proposal called for a study of epidemiology, preventive and social medicine, and "the medical control of society and the social control of medicine." Meanwhile, Buchanan tried to give order to the existing chaotic discussions that prevailed in medicine's public relations, hoping then that medicine might "find its point of entry into the new society . . . the Great Society of the modern world."

Second, in relation to the medical education of the day, *The Doctrine of Signatures* was written to persuade its readers that the Flexner reforms of a decade earlier had left medicine with "no genuine intellectual or scientific foundation." He maintained that Flexner's concept of scientific medicine also promoted anti-intellectualism and the "mysticism of fact" in medical schools; Buchanan observed, "In science when formal insights fail, only facts are trusted." As a liberal artist, he criticized the German notion of "science" as productive of an imbalance in the intellectual virtues—the arts of grammar, rhetoric, and logic—that together permit a science to become fully rational. The medical school of the future, vivified by the spirit of Galen, would provide the long-sought philosophy of science capable of surmounting the allied twin dangers of empiricism and mathematism. History has shown that the empirical sciences practiced by themselves too easily degenerate into the enslaving arts of technocracy and that the mathematical sciences too readily exert imperial claims over all the sciences, which can culminate in occult numerology or statistical mysticism. Hence by far exceeding Flexner's restrictive guidelines for professional education, Buchanan discerned that ultimately his theory of medicine necessarily incorporated the liberating Platonic ideal of education—"to know thyself."

This extraordinary admixture of philosophy, science, and

mathematics encompassed by *The Doctrine of Signatures* is given perspective in the realization that Buchanan viewed medicine first as a metaphysician, second as a semiotician, and always as a liberal artist. He was persevering in a search for intellectual freedom in the modern world then critically besieged by pragmatism, logical positivism, and scientism. The essential lines of his argument may be seen more clearly by disentangling those sources that form the matrix of his doctrine. Its metaphysical themes were derived principally from Aristotle's logic of demonstration and the semiotic themes from Galen's texts on physiology. His unique melding of concepts from the philosopher and the physician originate from his career as a teacher of the liberal arts and sciences. Also, in keeping with his innovative philosophy of mathematics of 1929, *Poetry and Mathematics,* he exposes the interrelations of mathematics with the physical sciences and encourages the convertibility of the disciplines of the *quadrivium* into those of the *trivium*—arithmetic and geometry, representing parallel grammars of measurement; music, a rhetoric reflecting the harmonies of the universe; and astronomy, a logic expressive of the constancy and regularity of the celestial bodies. To Buchanan, modern mathematics had lost or forsaken its foundations in the *trivium,* and the arts and sciences of medicine offered an opportunity to regain the unity of all seven liberal arts.

Buchanan's great expectation for *The Doctrine of Signatures,* summarized in the first six of his eight proposals for the profession, called for the creation of a new science of "physic, " a natural science or philosophy of nature discoursing on the human "organism as a whole. " This rational science and philosophy of nature is based on three universes of knowledge—the facts established by scientists in the realms of physics, phychobiology, sociology—with those truths organized by the philosopher or liberal artist according to three levels of understanding. This tripartite structure, an "architecture of ideas," gradually fabricated and subject to constant renovation is effected—through grammar providing a groundwork of empirical and practical truths; through rhetoric erecting a framework of rational and formal truths; and through logic completing and culminating the whole with durable, speculative truth. Buchanan insisted that such a study of humans as self-liberating artists would be the worthy heritage of a profession historically dedicated to intellectual freedom that now "has a record maximum of knowledge and a minimum of understanding." However, in the practice of medicine, art is manifested as the regulative, guiding principle in science because its operation—in the laboratory, through observation, hypothesis, and verification, and in the clinic, through diagnosis, prognosis, and therapy—imitates the order in nature and humanity. The doctor's artistry is to cooperate with the inherent restorative powers discoverable in nature and humanity.

Many aspects of Buchanan's doctrine are startlingly up-to-date. Recently, a reader was impressed by its relevance to clinical decision-making aided by computers. Programmers unwittingly have rediscovered Buchanan's cognitive "architecture," or a unified theory of cognition—"a generalized framework that makes learning, reason, and all the rest possible."[12] Another reviewer with an interest in medical education remarked on the possibilities of the "transformational" medical grammar suggested by Buchanan for effecting a revolution similar to the consequences of Chomsky's linguistic theories on the teaching of languages.[13] Buchanan's final proposal, the establishment of a permanent board to critique and codify medical knowledge as it might affect public policy, remained unfulfilled until 1970 when the Institute of Medicine was formed under the National Academy of Sciences. Nevertheless, many now would opt for a separate, independent National Academy of Medicine to achieve that goal.[14] Furthermore, in 1988 the author of *Medical Semiotics* described Buchanan's work as providing the impetus to develop an integration of the sciences with themselves and with medicine.[15] Without question his terse commentaries on current intellectual prejudices sprinkled throughout *The Doctrine of Signatures* awaken the reader to new possibilities for thought and reflection.

In substance *The Doctrine of Signatures* is a metaphysical work that condenses more profound insights into the philosophy of medicine than any comparable work on the subject. Using basic, straightforward language, Buchanan has outlined a pioneering program of studies for future generations of medical professionals. Because major issues in the socialization of medicine continue to fester and Flexner's ideals for medical education still dominate the curriculum, his message is still pertinent fifty years later. His favorite aphorism, "medicine is the science of the soul and science is the medicine of the soul," points toward Buchanan's goal of a comprehensive doctrine uniting the liberal, laboratory, medical, and useful arts under a new philosophy, a rational science of nature and humanity.

NOTES

1. Edmund D. Pellegrino, "The Clinical Arts and the Arts of the Word," *The Pharos* (Fall 1981): 2–8.

2. Personal communication with the author.

3. Plato, *The Dialogues of Plato*, 11th ed., trans. B. Jowett. (New York: Random House, 1937), 491.

4. E. Lederman, *Philosophy and Medicine*, rev. ed. (Great Britain, 1986), 19.

5. Eric J. Cassell, "Ideas in Conflict," *Daedalus* (Spring 1986): 20.

6. Harris L. Coulter, *Divided Legacy: A History of the Schism in Medical Thought*, vol. 1 (Washington, D.C.: Wehawken Books, 1975), 506.

7. Thure von Uexküll, "Semiotics and Medicine," in *Semiotica* (Amsterdam: Mouton, 1982), 205.

8. Fielding H. Garrison, *An Introduction to the History of Medicine*, 4th ed. (Philadelphia: W. B. Saunders, 1929), 796.

9. Odin W. Anderson, *Health Services of the United States* (Ann Arbor: Health Administration Press, 1985), 96–97.

10. Morris Fishbein, editorial, *Journal of the American Medical Association* 99, no. 24 (10 Dec. 1932): 2034–35

11. John Deely, *Introducing Semiotic: Its History and Doctrine* (Bloomington: Indiana University Press, 1982), 145.

12. M. Mitchell Waldrop, "Soar: A Unified Theory of Cognition," *Science*, 15 July 1988, 296.

13. Personal communication with the author.

14. Editorial, *Journal of the American Medical Association*, 260, no. 14 (15 July 1988): 2105.

15. Eugen Baer, *Medical Semiotics* (Lanham, Md.: University Press of America, 1988), 1–2.

INTRODUCTION

In the writing of this book the dominating interest has been in the freedom of speculation. There are many signs that speculation is not free. I am not thinking primarily of the social and political restraints on free thought that are appearing all over the world, but rather of the doubts and fears within the individual thinker himself. We doubt the efficacy of the intellectual process and we fear its consequences. I find this doubt and fear in my fellow philosophers ; I have found it in myself as I have written this book. I believe it has bad consequences for the more generally accepted empirical and analytic modes of thought.

The fearless defence of civil liberties, essential and admirable as it may be, does not touch the inner sources from which free thought flows. Civil liberties are permissive but not enabling, and it is not surprising that some have concluded that they are stultifying. I have chosen to consider a profession and a subject-matter in which these remarks on liberty are amply illustrated, namely medicine. Here is a profession which has fought and won the good battle for freedom of thought ; in fact throughout European history it has continually fought and won that battle, even when individual medical men lacked the aids of explicit organization. On the other hand, there have been times when freedom to think has become freedom not to think, and freedom of thought has resulted in freedom from thought. I realize that there are many reasons for this default, and when there are not genuine reasons there are many practical excuses. We hear a rather full array of such reasons and excuses at present. Contemporary medicine, however, shows what might be called an excess of speculative energy. Intellectually and imaginatively it is rearing and plunging to go. It stands at the head of the natural sciences, and does not know which way to go. It has a record maximum of knowledge and a minimum of understanding, to say nothing of practical and philosophical wisdom. It has art, and wonders if it has science. It is suffering from an imbalance of intellectual virtues, and in this it is typical of many organizations bent on intellectual enterprises.

I am here offering two ancient traditional remedies, whose apparent novelty is due only to our forgetfulness : symbols and demonstration. Let there be no misunderstanding to begin with. I am not prescribing this or that set of symbols ; on the contrary I am prescribing certain exercises, the liberal arts and sciences, for the heightening and strengthening of our response and operations with whatever symbols our going affairs present to us. Again, I am not making demonstrations ; that would be egregiously impertinent in view of the issues that have grown out of the present state of knowledge in medicine. I am merely suggesting the kind of terms, tools, and techniques that would make demonstration possible, and the place and function that demonstration might hold in modern medicine, by showing these things in Galenic medicine. Given the means I believe the medical profession would dare and do much, not only for itself, but for other professions and for all of us, in the way of speculation.

I have introduced symbols in medical dress under the title, the Doctrine of Signatures. This doctrine for various reasons has the air of a myth about it. It has often been given a mythical statement, and in that form is a powerful piece of medical rhetoric. Viewed from this angle it is the expression of our vague yearnings for an integral medical science. In sober language it says that medical knowledge and skill consists in seeing the connections between symptoms and remedies. It is invoked when we say that the symptoms of malaria indicate quinine as the remedy, or when we say that quinine is the specific for malaria. These judgments have some rational content. It is perhaps easier to see the signatures themselves when there is a minimum of explicit rational content as when the extract of the heartshaped leaves of the fox-glove is called the specific for angina pectoris. This is a classic illustration and it is usually cited to show the primitive imagination correlating shapes of organs and shapes of herbs by magical impulse. Actually it is the mnemonic distillate of what must have been considerable experience. It is a better illustration of empiricism in medicine. Two things should be noted about it : its truth value is not zero : its truth value can be increased by more knowledge. However, there is an illusion connected with the latter point. More judgments of the same kind seem to increase knowledge, but actually they do not unless they involve an increment of rational content. It is to avoid this illusion and to insure the increment of rational content that the liberal and liberating arts are employed. They move symbols about and adjust their relative positions so that rational content and science may be introduced. Modern empirical sciences are the descendants of the liberal arts, and the modern diagnostic arts apply them to the signatures of disease and remedies, but the results in unambiguous indications of specifics are relatively disappointing, and the contributions to genuine medical science are even more disappointing. I am therefore accusing modern scientific medicine of elaborate empiricism and of anti-intellectualism, and I am prescribing the doctrine of signatures for contemplation and the original liberal arts for the exercise of our weak symbolic faculties. Such practice should strengthen the intellectual virtues.

There is a great deal of pious talk about the unity and wholeness of the organism, and the understanding of that is set up as the next objective of medical science. At the same time the well-tried but less well-known intellectual terms, tools, and techniques are eschewed because of what seems to many their abortive success in mathematics and mechanics. Since Kant, demonstration in any but these sciences has been doubted and feared. On the other hand, it must be obvious that a unified organism cannot be understood without a unified intellect, and that the unity of the intellect can express itself only in demonstration. The disuse of demonstration in the biological and medical sciences has led to the atrophy and paralysis of the understanding. The unity of the understanding is now sought in mysticism and statistics. For this I, as philosopher who rushes in where physicians fear to tread, propose a consideration of the terms of ancient analysis and speculation, form and matter.

The power of speculation depends on a unity that can comprehend diversity ; the phrase arouses a quick antipathy in us because we have so often been thwarted in our attempts to achieve its ideal. Again the mathematician alone seems to be able to sustain the intellectual effort that it invokes. But his secret is that he has retained the ancient distinction of form and matter in his new terminology. Functions and variables are forms ; values and constants are matter. Their distinction and combination are the essentials of mathematics.

Plato, Aristotle, and Galen found and established the demonstrative power of form and matter in biological and medical science, and I have tried to show how they did it. Its rediscovery and re-establishment in modern signatures would invigorate and show the way for our thwarted speculative energies.

I am indebted to Mortimer Adler and Richard McKeon for being good companions in the larger speculative enterprise ; to Everett Martin who has allowed us to lecture on these matters at the People's Institute, New York ; to Doctor Henry Sigerist and Doctor Owsei Temkin who gave me the freedom of the Institute of the History of Medicine; to Doctors Chesney, Weed, Longcope and Meyer who let me see medicine in operation in the anatomy room and the clinical wards of the Johns Hopkins Medical School ; to Doctor Ludwig Kast whose friendship and aid encouraged me to finish this statement ; and to Ethel S. Dummer, whose wisdom and humanity have tempered the doctrine that I have tried to present.

THE DOCTRINE OF SIGNATURES

CHAPTER I

THE documents in the history of medicine show a persistent concern with the influence of philosophy on medical thought and practice. Feeling runs high, the issues are varied, and the dialectical conclusions are regularly incorporated in the dogmatic holdings of the medical schools and cults. This historical perspective may lead the dialectician or the medical student to one or the other of two conclusions : either that medicine sets up its professional shop on foundations borrowed from current philosophical opinion ; or that philosophy periodically rebuilds itself by generalizing medical knowledge. Both these conclusions have a specious truth, but the accusing tone of their statements arouses the suspicion that they are the sort of conclusions that hide and prevent the proper statement of the question.

Supposing that the question concerns the proper relation of medicine and philosophy, we may certainly propose other possible patterns in which their relation or relations may be found. It would be pleasant to find a pattern in which there would be many organic relations between the two, each serving as a route of communication and at the same time marking the line at which some division of labour can be recognized and respected. I believe that there is such a pattern and that it would be useful in any attempt to clarify the two fields of thought.

Perhaps the best introduction to it is to be found in the Platonic dialogue which goes by the name of the *Charmides*. This is one of the earlier dialogues. It has a very charming dramatic movement ; it contains the famous Socratic aphorisms in more than their usual seductive setting, and it manages by skilful intellectual obstetrics to deliver several minds of infant ideas. These ideas innocently enough appear to add to our understanding of the moral virtue, temperance, but they suddenly grow up to make sophisticated suggestions for the improvement of medicine, and we finally realize that they have grown old and a bit mystical about such revered matters as the acquisition of truth and the achievement of the good life. In short, the *Charmides* is the earliest proposal in European literature of the issues between medicine and philosophy. A bit of detail will make this clear.

Socrates, in the course of doing his round of scrutiny of Athenian institutions, has come to a gymnasium, where health, love, and athletics are pursued in a lively social atmosphere. It is an Athenian institution because its doings are always completed with good talk ; Socrates would not be there if this sort of completion were lacking. It is made clear in Plato's account of the conversation that a certain Charmides is the centre of both the doings and the talk. Socrates immediately wants to meet and talk with Charmides, and their mutual friends start manœuvres for a graceful introduction should the occasion arrive. Presently Charmides comes in, and it is reported that he has a headache. Socrates decides to play the role of physician, on one condition, that he shall be allowed to use an incantation as well as the usual arts of diagnosis and prescription. The introduction is made, the condition is accepted by Charmides, and the consultation begins with talk about diet and exercise. But the questions soon become general and drift to the discussion of temperance as the health of the soul. It turns out that Socrates is asking an expert in temperate living about the nature of his accomplishments and has made an ironic application of the two Delphic inscriptions : Nothing too much, and Know thyself. Charmides, without realizing the irony, has admitted that Knowledge is Virtue and that he himself is ignorant. Socrates thus makes his customary diagnosis, *ignorance*, and points out that the only remedy is knowledge. There follows a search for the specific remedy for the vice of intemperance, and it at length appears to be an incantation invoking a science of all the sciences, by which any given empirical science would be able to transform its subject matter into genuine knowledge. The headache appears trivial beside the defect which has been detected in the soul, and the medical man appears in Socrates who joins the patient in seeking a rational remedy.

This is a complicated dialectical tangle for the presentation of medical and philosophical problems, but it sets the tradition in which these problems are still discussed. It may be interesting to see what lies between it and our modern tangles of laboratories, clinics, and medical associations, which do without philosophy.

The proposal of a science of the sciences is, of course, a riddle characteristically Delphic in its manifold significances. It has ever since played the role of catch-question, and made fools of many bright answerers. Any beginning student of philosophy during and since the nineteenth century would naïvely assume that Plato was here proposing that philosophy itself is the science of the sciences, and would further assume that the middle ages would have as easily and unquestioningly proposed theology. Plato would have made Socrates accept these answers as mere opinions for further scrutiny if they had been made at the end of the *Charmides*, and the result would have been that both theology and philosophy would have become learned ignorances seeking a still higher science. The fact is that any science becomes a learned ignorance as soon as it thinks of itself as the science of all other sciences. The teaching of the *Charmides* is contained in the Delphic motto, Know thyself. When it is addressed to a science, or, as in the case of medicine, to a profession which has science at the base of its arts, it means that any given science should take itself as a science among sciences and seek a science of these sciences, at the same time holding its position of responsibility for still lower sciences. Only thus does it come to know itself in a wise and critical way, and obey the other dictum, Nothing too much.

But this is still a riddle or an incantation, and the only time in western history when it became effective in application was in the medieval university. An expansion of it in terms of the curriculum of the medieval university is necessary to its understanding. It is not misleading to take the *Charmides* as the original statement of the proper functions of the university faculty of medicine.

The medieval university was not merely concerned with the acquisition of knowledge as is the modern university, which estimates its value by the amount of research it turns out. It was concerned with teaching and the necessary conditions for clarifying and protecting an intellectual tradition from its constant dangers of degradation and misuse. Thus the Liberal Arts were sharply distinguished from the Black Arts and were taught to every student before he was allowed to go on to professional studies. A master of arts had the training and knowledge to enable him to avoid the subtle snares and pitfalls which the perpetuation and advance of any department of knowledge must risk. The technical arts and their practice always threaten the liberal arts and it is the ever present bastard combinations of these that are called Black Arts.

The persistent attempt in the medieval university to communicate the liberal arts to its students is like animal evolution at the stage when internal skeletons displaced external skeletons ; the Liberal Arts were taught in the hope that internal understanding would take the place of the external social defence of dogma and right opinion. The attempt to work this change in mentality was amazingly successful in some cases, but it is not surprising that it failed in general and that we are still wavering between the Inquisition on the one hand and liberalism without art on the other.

The liberal arts were seven in number and they were divided into two groups, the trivium and the quadrivium.

These two groups have the same formal distinctions within them and for the purposes of this essay only the distinctions within the trivium will be emphasized. The trivium deals with the gross distinctions in the modes of signification that are to be found in the use of symbols. The quadrivium deals with those finer distinctions which are necessary for the special use of symbols that we have in mathematics. The distinction, making of the trivium and the quadrivium is the feature in medieval thought that is often referred to by modern writers as logic-chopping and endless argumentation. Both these epithets are just, but neither logic-chopping nor endless argument should be objected to by moderns who become unintentionally tangled in their own symbols in simple conversational discourse.

Grammar is the first element of the trivium but the term grammar itself is subject to analysis according to the trivium, and it should therefore not be presented as a simple term. It properly refers to at least three different things. In the first place it refers to the art of writing, according to its obvious etymology. Writing in its simplest meaning is a process made up of operations by which elementary concrete units such as letters or marks are given positions and related to each other. Grammar then in its first mode of signifying means the art of writing.

Grammar in its second mode of signifying is the science of writing, that is the analytical account of the elements and the operations that enter into the practice of the art. This is very close to our ordinary school-book meaning for grammar according to which we classify letters into consonants, vowels, mutes, liquids, and sibilants, or words into nouns, verbs, adjectives, and adverbs, and then state the rules for their combination, letters into words, and words into sentences. This second meaning for grammar is somewhat complicated by the fact that there is a very special grammatical art involved in constructing the science of grammar, in other words there is a writing technique in making a grammatical analysis. However, this should not confuse anyone if it is remembered that the so-called construction of a science is not a science itself but rather an historical accident that happens to a science which was in some sense there before the construction and remains after the art has done its work.

This leads to the third meaning for grammar, namely the product of the art after the operations are completed. There will be at least two kinds of such products, one the product of a given practice of the art, namely a piece of writing, say a sentence or an essay, and the other a product of the scientific analysis, a dictionary or a work of grammar as we understand it, say a book called English Grammar. Both these can be called grammars when they are thought of as instruments, as when we say that a stylist like Proust or Joyce has given us a new grammar or language which we may imitate or practise. Proust and Joyce are grammatical artists and have produced grammars just as truly as Jespersen has been a grammatical scientist and given us an English grammar, although the senses in which they have done grammar are quite different. In this case as in many others in the trivium we have a difficult time deciding whether we shall make up or hunt up different terms for the different meanings or whether we shall face the real state of affairs and admit that all words have different modes of signifying, which must be distinguished and yet related closely if we are going to be successful in discourse.

This problem is somewhat simplified if we accept the medieval terms for these distinctions. The terms have an accidental pictorial value also which aids our understanding of symbols in general. The medieval grammarians spoke of the impositions that words have received, uses that have been put upon them (impono). A word has first imposition when it is used to signify or point out something else, as when I say " table " and mean the thing I am writing on. A word has second imposition when it is used to refer to itself, as when I say " table is a noun " ; I am then making " table " refer to itself as a word. One can see that second impositions are useful in constructing a science of grammar and that first impositions are useful in the practice of writing or in the art of grammar, and that these impositions will be found in a variety of combinations. The notion of an imposition helps a great deal when we see that it calls attention to the functions of symbols, that is to refer beyond themselves in various ways in the many possible modes of signifying. In fact when this is recognized it is important to note that the elements of a grammar either in the artistic sense or the scientific sense are concrete things taken by themselves. Taken with their appropriate operations of combination they are called notations, instruments of noting. Grammar then is the art of noting, the science of noting, and its products are notations. There is the suggestion here that grammar will easily extend beyond the narrow and familiar arts that deal with words to include any medium or material that is used for noting, for instance scientific instruments. This will later be developed in the discussion of scientific method.

At certain periods grammar has been the art of reading. When this has been so there has usually been associated with the art the scholar whose professional business is to read documents or texts and to interpret them. In some sense this is the inverse of writing, in which there is a subject-matter either concrete or abstract which is being noted ; in reading there is the notation and a subject matter either concrete or abstract which is being extracted from it. Very often the scholar is concerned with the reading of a document or text which has been written in a comparatively unknown language, and even in a known language there is often the necessity of interpreting an unusual style. Whenever this is the case there is a choice of a more familiar grammar or language into which the original is translated. In translation the grammatical art and science must become more refined and complicated in order to overcome an initial psychological difficulty.

Translation is, of course, a kind of combination of reading and writing, reading from a text and writing a new text. The two texts must have some kind of correspondence, though the materials or elements of the two may be very different. This argues a common form which may lie only on some high level of generality in the two grammars involved, and successful translation will depend upon the subtlety with which the grammatical sciences of the two texts have been understood. A deficient training in grammar in one's own language may make different texts or styles untranslatable, or two persons with different styles unintelligible to one another, even when they are acquainted with the same subject-matters. Many of the problems in the higher branches of grammar are occasioned by difficulties of translation.

Already in discussing translation I have brought in considerations that are essentially matters of the next art of the trivium, namely rhetoric. Rhetoric, as literally understood, is the art of speaking, though its customary meaning is public speaking with the aim of persuasion. The chief reason that it has this connection with speaking lies in a peculiarity of speaking as distinguished from writing and reading. Writing and reading have no narrow time limits ; they can be done successfully both slow and fast. Speaking on the other hand has narrower time limits if it is to escape the failures that come from boredom, weak attention, the inarticulateness of rapid speech, or the slow mentality of the hearer. Both reader and writer can pick up loose ends at their leisure, but the speaker must risk everything on one recital. These exigencies, though not met in the formal use of symbols, do indirectly impose demands on the conventional uses of language, many of whose corresponding elaborate formal devices are then discovered to be of great use in writing.

Most of the rhetorical devices did not begin, as is usually said, in ornamentation, but rather in the need for condensation and expansion in length of discourse. Condensations and expansions are usually accomplished by figures of speech,[1] and they are the traditional elementary units for rhetorical analysis. On examination figures

[1] See *Symbolic Distance*. Kegan Paul, 1932.

of speech turn out to be implicit translations, or speaking in two languages at once. It seems that translation is most effective rhetorically when the laboured detail of correspondence is concealed, as for instance when the laboured Anglo-Saxon paraphrase of a Latin word is given up for a new Anglicized Latin word. The resulting contagion and conflict of two languages has at first a disruptive effect, but the chaos is soon ordered by mutual concessions in the figurative and fictional use of words. Elizabethan English was the cure for the chaos following the introduction of Latin words. The figures then invented helped greatly to make English a rich and rhetorically versatile language.

The organic patterns that lie back of figures of speech are analogies. From the grammatical approach the analogy appears to be the placing of the elements of two languages side by side to show the common form that their disparate material elements have. When this is done for the purpose of translation one of these analogues is taken as archetypal text and the other becomes the secondary or derivative of the former. The second appears then to be an expansion of the first by a kind of mirroring. If their positions are reversed for the purpose of checking the translation, and the checking is successful, the two languages are seen as equally adequate expressions of a common form or meaning, although the individual traits of the two languages may still render one preferable for specific occasions which present practical peculiarities. The formal properties of the analogy are seen only when the two analogues seem equally adequate and the translation and counter-translation can be easily seen. Good linguists can play between two languages in this way, but the ordinary person with the mother tongue will have to find his analogies within one conventional language between two styles or two technical terminologies.   One of the mysterious virtues of training in the older classical languages was the feeling for words that resulted from it ; it was often a feeling for the hidden analogies that an analytical study of grammar gives its devotees.

There is no reason why a good training within one conventional language should not be coupled with a clear analytic grammar with the resulting sensitivity to figures of speech and their analogical matrices.   The training would consist in the practice of translation of one style or technical terminology into another within the same conventional language.   The modern divisions of the sciences with their special terminologies afford ample diversities of such sub-languages and their grammars.   If such a training were given there would very likely be objection from the scientist, because students would discover that supposedly literal propositions in science are highly metaphorical and sometimes even allegorical.   One scientific language has grown out of another and all of them out of a linguistic tradition, so that translation has done its disruptive and synthetic work even in technical formulae.   Perhaps the scientist would discover that the danger of figurative language is not directly consequent on its presence, but rather on the oversight involved in supposing that any language including his own is not figurative.

Supposing that the figures are recognized and their corresponding analogies brought to light we can see how rhetorical devices are invented. A given piece of discourse is expanded by the addition of its analogue in other terms. Insight into the adequacy of the translation and the analogical pattern within which it moves will allow one to substitute terms from one analogue to the other and we shall have the basis for the whole range of metaphorical shorthand propositions. Likewise the given discourse can be put into a larger context in which it will appear as part of a larger analogical matrix in which there may be more than two analogues, and more than two terms in each analogue. Then we can choose allegories and fables from the pattern, or the whole pattern may be represented by one word, as when we refer in biology to evolution, which is rhetorically speaking a story told in temporal terms reflecting the static terms of the classification of organisms. A language itself is a kind of dramatic allegory in which letters and words are the actors, manipulated like marionettes by writer, reader, and speaker to reflect each other and the things that are being talked about analogically.

Rhetoric is the art of using two languages to say the same thing. This means that there will be two grammars, one for each of the languages, and that the two or more grammars will have enough in common to justify their correlation and use in a single discourse. The simplest case of this will be seen in the analogy of four terms where one ratio or analogue will correspond to another ratio or analogue by virtue of like relations between the members of the pairs. Window is to house what eye is to mind. It is possible here to translate from the window-house language to the eye-mind language, and in this context we can say that window signifies eye and house signifies mind, or vice versa. Or, to return to grammar, we can say that the first imposition of window is eye, and likewise the first imposition of house is mind. The second impositions are illustrated if we say that eye is the first member of the analogy of which mind is the last. If we wish, we can give a name to the common thing of which they are both speaking, namely, Johnnie's power to learn by observation. But I believe this interpretation will seem restricted and arbitrary. We feel a generality in an analogy, or in any derived figure of speech which makes any concrete application appear slightly ridiculous. There is more in the analogy than four nominal terms will account for.

This brings us to a tangle in the modes of signifying which has tried men's minds and hearts and driven them to the most daring creative heights as well as the most destructive manias. As far as the liberal arts are concerned, we may calmly proceed with the disentanglement of a complicated pattern of confluent lines of reference and let the metaphysics of nominalism, realism, and conceptualism await the issue of the battle of the arts. First let it be clear just how the formal grammatical structure of the analogy has let in this generality.

It comes in first by the translator's discovery that there are at least two ways of saying the same thing, perhaps by using two recognized languages or by using two terminologies within the same language. Over against these two artificially constructed grammars there is supposedly a concrete situation which is being named or described and analysed by both. But it is often discovered that there is another concrete situation which the same grammatical formulae describe. It appears that the two concrete situations have the same relation to each other that the two grammars have, and we can speak of a translation from one situation to the other. This is much like the notion of spatial translation of figures in geometry. It seems also that the original linguistic description is itself a translation from concrete to artificial verbal language and that the translation is reversible, as it is in the experimental verification of a scientific formula. But this translatability in languages was recognized as due to a common grammatical form in the two versions. There seems to be no reason in the arts to deny that there is a common grammatical form in the two concrete situations, and that it is our recognition of this that is expressed in the assertion in the case of the similarity of the two situations that they have the same form, or that they belong to the same class of things. Their differences argue grammatical differences also, and on analysis we find that the situations are made of similar things which still have layers of relative similarities and differences as far as we wish to uncover them. It is this common grammatical form that has puzzled those metaphysicians who have attended to the endless similarities and differences in things.

We are here standing at the point where rhetoric changes grammar into logic, the third of the arts of the trivium. The master of the liberal arts, who cannot therefore be the slave of one alone, will easily admit that there are forms in things, ideas or abstract concepts in minds, and essences which have being independently of any time-space instances, and it is these that have given artificial discourse its grammatical forms. To the nominalist who stands on good grammatical ground when he says that these common forms are made up of the similar uses to which we put words in talking about similars, the master of the arts answers that words are words, notations are notations, only when the ways they are used express abstract forms, whether these are explicitly recognized or not. In logic it is well to call them universals. It is these by virtue of which the members of classes have common properties and similarities which allow them to be divided and subdivided according to identities and differences and arranged in analogical patterns.

But it is not only regarding this problem of classes that the master of all the arts can inform and enlighten the mere grammarian. There is the persistent problem of what is called height, elevation, or sublimity in good discourse that he can explain. There is a reversal or conversion in good discourse which corresponds to the turning point in tragedy. Suddenly everything said goes to a different level and is transfigured. When the shift is felt, but not understood, it is called supernatural, and is said to awaken a sense of glory. It is the ghost that haunts poetry.

The trivial explanation of it is founded on a distinction between the intentions of terms. This distinction falls within the first imposition on words. According to first imposition words refer beyond themselves to other things. The intentions distinguish different kinds of things signified by the same sign. There are on one hand individual concrete objects and aggregates or classes of these objects. But now the master of the arts points out that there are also universals. When terms in the first imposition refer to concrete objects or groups of them the terms have first intention. When they refer to universals they have second intention. The reversal or conversion in sublime discourse happens when speech or writing reveals the second intentions. The mystery is due to the fact that terms may have both first and second intention, and when they do, we feel the ambiguity due to the presence of the ghostly universals in the concrete objects. The moment of discovery of a law in science brings the same sense of elevation.

There is an interesting and dangerous incidence that the intentions have upon terms as used in the second imposition, when words are made to refer to themselves. It gives rise to unrecognized paradoxes and nonsense when it does not openly mislead into confusion. A word is used in second imposition when it refers to itself, but there is involved in this a curious confluence of the modes of signification. For instance, I may count the times that the word " dog " occurs on a given page and may give the result by saying " dog " occurs twenty-two times on this page. In this case the paradox arises in trying to answer this question : Is the word " dog " an individual object, a class, or a universal? The correct answer from the point of view of the trivial artist is that, like all other words, it has all these references and they should and must be distinguished. The marks on the paper are the thing talked about as well as the notation used in the talk, and both of these represent in their mutual relations the class of dogs and the universal dog. This is really no more complex than any other case of the use of words although this case forces distinctions which are not obvious. Perhaps this example will show why the adjective " trivial " arose from the noun " trivium ", and why finally triviality spread its net of signification until it caught the trivium itself.

When rhetoric has laid bare the structures that lie at the basis of its various arts, in other words is aware of itself in terms of translations, analogies and figures of speech, it may turn to sophistical dialectic. It will by this time have become sophisticated about universals, and the sophistical rhetorician will be able to fit symbols together on the threads of ideas and fabricate long arguments within which the laws of logic that govern the subsumption of classes and the marvellous ways of the syllogism will support imagination, persuade listeners, and fool the orator himself. It is not only the professional public man who indulges in this kind of trivial art, but the modern scientist also shows the same romantic disposition. Actually the sophist is at heart a very puzzled man, and if he takes a political or a scientific holiday he will at least wonder if there is not a better use for his rhetorical skill. If he does not turn into a popular writer he may discover the proper end for his rhetorical means, namely the use of his devices in the service of abstract ideas. For the rhetorician of well-known reputation, the juggler of words and arguments, ideas are the means to his end of persuasion and entertainment ; to the rhetorician, who has reached the insights of logic, ideas are the ends to be sought and figures of speech are the subtle and elegant ways by which the connections and consistencies of ideas are revealed. There are systems of ideas that can be grasped only by very involved literary devices, or possibly by very complicated machinery which has been put to the uses of precise knowledge. Then the laws of logic and the rules of the syllogism are the necessary tools for the refinement of technical and professional knowledge. The finest accomplishments in this art rest upon special accomplishments in the other arts of the trivium and have been reached, I believe, only in medieval logic and modern mathematics, where the notational means and the rhetorical patterns have been worked over and over again until they have reached a high degree of elegance and efficiency.

It should have become clear that the trivial arts are interpenetrative. The necessity to begin somewhere forced the first description of grammar into a narrow mode of signification in which it appeared as independent of rhetoric and logic. It would be unfortunate if it were left in that mode alone. The rules of operation in grammar conceal their logical nature as long as we are dealing with symbols as mere notations. The notion that words are names conceals the radically analogical nature of notations. Actually grammatical things move in an atmosphere of rhetoric and logic from which they take their life. Notations are imitations of things : the thing as known imitates the mode of notation by which it is known. Grammatical elements are analogues of things, though the subtlety of linguistic operations often conceals this. Similarly grammatical forms are shadows of ideas, and they bear witness to their logical affiliations by their constancy and invariance under such transformations as translation and elevation. This leads to the cardinal principle of the trivium and all the liberal arts, namely that each symbol has all the references that I have distinguished under their medieval names, first and second impositions, and first and second intentions. The arts by which they are distinguished and organized in discourse are obviously important. Discourse produces many confusions of falsity and truth, fiction and fact, when its subtleties are neglected as they have been for the last four or five hundred years.

The quadrivium was studied and practised after the student's thorough mastery of the trivium, partly because it was thought to be more difficult and partly because it was the extension of the principles and distinctions made by the trivium in ordinary discourse to the mediums proper to mathematics. Until fairly recently modern mathematicians went their independent ways confident in their proficiency in their specialized notations, but there has always been an unapproved occult practice of mathematics running along beside the academic and professional tradition. Sometimes this occult practice consists merely in the applications of mathematics, as in astrology, alchemy, numerology, accounting, and statistics, but there is periodically a kind of occult disease that strikes deep into pure mathematics itself and it comes from the mathematical magicians, the calculators and operationalists. Recently the disease has become acute and there have been heart-breaking attempts to diagnose and cure it. The attempts of mathematicians and philosophers to look into the foundations of mathematics have had curious results. Sometimes they have announced

the decay of these foundations and have tried to rebuild
a less ambitious edifice on new and smaller foundations.
Very often they have only succeeded in adding to the
magic. It seems that they have not been masters in the
arts of the trivium, for it is there that the distinctions are
made which clarify any field which is suffering occultation.
I am not saying that the task is simple or easily accomplished ; mathematics has gone very far forward even in
the last hundred years without benefit of trivial criticism.
I am saying that nothing less than the trivium will suffice.

I do not wish to go into this matter at this point, but
I can suggest from the medieval background some of the
things that are missing in the philosophy of mathematics
at present, and that will serve my purpose here, which is
to show the preliminary disciplines that were thought
necessary in undergraduate training in the medieval
university. The quadrivium consisted of arithmetic,
geometry, music and astronomy. Arithmetic provided a
mathematical grammar wherein numbers were parts of
speech and their laws of combination described accepted
notational procedures. Geometry is a parallel grammar
having its independent elements and rules of operation,
which for instance in Euclid are carried out chiefly by
ruler and compass. But before geometry had proceeded
very far, it fell back on the rhetorical device of translation,
in this case into arithmetic. In fact the two arts,
arithmetic and geometry, developed side by side and their
terminologies still show their analogical and figurative
relations ; for instance, we still have square numbers.
Geometry as earth measurement goes still farther into
rhetorical modes, seeing the analogies between distances,

lines, and numbers, and giving the results of surveying in concrete numbers. However, music is the rhetoric of mathematics in the most thorough-going sense. Starting with the discovery of the numerical and geometrical expressions for musical intervals, it covers in the developed quadrivium the whole field of precise measurement. Its analogies and figures of mathematical speech were very early wondered at as the music of the spheres. Modern mathematical physics very worthily carries on the romantic tradition, Newton's law of gravitation defining the intervals for modern celestial compositions. Music as understood in the quadrivium is the magic bridge by which the non-mathematical world can be reduced to harmony, and the forms which are so clearly expressed in mathematical notation can be abstracted and transferred to the notations of the trivium. Thus wave-lengths which were first found in water are next found in trigonometric formulae and then by suitable experimentation are rediscovered in colour, x-rays, and radio waves.

But as soon as the stage is reached where formulae are separable from proportions and analogies we are again elevated to the level of logic, which because of the regularities of the orbits of the planets and the sempiternal revolution of the heavens is called astronomy in the mathematical arts. If algebra had been better known in the middle ages it would have displaced the name astronomy, which in modern thought really corresponds to music in the quadrivium. Astronomy of the old quadrivium would to-day study the invariant functions in mathematics and their consistencies as revealed in the differential calculus and modern group theory. Again passing from arithmetic to astronomy through geometry and music we have discovered in mathematics the two impositions and the two intentions of the trivium; likewise we find that the mathematical arts and sciences are not like beads on a string, but are interpenetrative patterns consisting of lines of reference following the trivial modes of signifying. Theory of functions and group theory in modern mathematics, which would belong to astronomy, often appear as combinatorial arts on the grammatical level, and in their succeeding trivial revelations send out illuminating rays on the figures in geometry and the natures that make up the physical world.

Modern mathematics has in its own madcap ways spun webs of fine distinctions and covered itself with many veils, and if I can judge from my own amateur attempts, the disentanglement of these webs and the unveiling of quadrivial mysteries is the best route for rediscovering the subtleties and niceties of the lost trivium. The analogies between the two afford royal roads for the necessary pilgrimage back to clear speech and ordered thinking in any subject-matter.

Perhaps so much will serve to describe the main principles and suggest the essential atmosphere of the medieval university, and in turn that will throw light on the riddle Socrates was announcing when he proposed to treat Charmides with an incantation as well as with efficient remedies. Diagnosis and therapeutics are embedded in a verbal and rational context, and if they are to be used with intelligence and fitness, the nature of that context must be ascertained and kept in view.

Hence the question of the science of sciences must be raised. The interpretation of the incantation that Socrates was proposing for all future medicine in the *Charmides* is to be found in the application of the trivium to the symbols of medicine, both in their artistic uses and in their scientific modes of signifying.

CHAPTER II

AT this point I might go on to the description of the content of the graduate curriculum in medicine as it, together with law and theology, formed the graduate curriculum of the medieval university. This would show how medicine becomes a science in the ordinary sense of natural science. That will come later. For the present purpose I should like to make some applications of the trivium to modern scientific method as a step towards its more specific application to medicine in the doctrine of signatures.

In the introductory chapter of his *History of European Thought in the Nineteenth Century*, Theodor Merz lays special emphasis on the change of meaning that the term " science " underwent when it migrated from France to Germany and England. In France it had meant any body of knowledge having those rational properties that make strict deduction possible. In Germany it meant a set of compendent propositions that cover a field of knowledge. In England it meant any body of propositions that generalize a collection of facts. In France the ideal science was mechanics, in Germany history, in England natural history. Roughly these divisions in culture divide the arts of the trivium between the three countries and argue that Frenchmen have a flair for logic, Germans

25

a flair for rhetoric, and Englishmen a flair for grammar. Their failures in science point to their respective single-track pursuits of the separate intellectual arts.

History has always shown this separate and kaleido-scopic application of the trivium, and one can characterize intellectual epochs by giving the order in which the trivium was taught.   The Greeks in general put logic or dialectic last and understood the other two arts as steps preliminary and subsidiary to the end.   The Alexandrians put grammar at the top of the educational ladder and turned out learned readers and commentators on texts. The Romans held rhetoric in highest esteem and put logic on the level of legal pleading.   At some point in the middle ages, probably around the middle of the thirteenth century, there were at least a few persons of learning who held the three arts in equal esteem and appear to be equally skilled in each ; the much slandered dialectician could speak the trivial dialects smoothly and impartially. Since then the history of philosophical systems mirrors the modern battle of the arts.   It seems that the Jesuits began teaching the quadrivium first and letting the trivium follow as best it could.   The rationalism of the seventeenth century represented a logical interest in mathematics, confused the trivium with theology and fought against what rationalists thought was the obscurantism of both.   The discoveries of the physicists were made as applications of mathematics and finally measurement took the field.   There was a resurgence of the trivium in the classical humanists, and the story from then on has been the conflict between devotees of these very closely complementary arts each losing its own virtues by exclusive cultivation of its own independent powers. At present all have sunk to the level of grammars without rules, or, as the laboratory scientist would have it, facts without hypotheses. This is more particularly true of the English-speaking world. Continental cultures do not so easily lose their pasts.

The great advances in the last three hundred years are usually celebrated as the successive triumphs of empiricism in science. It may seem absurd to say that this is the latest battle cry of the grammarians, but it is connected with the next previous battle cry which argues for the retention of Greek and Latin grammar in the school curriculum on the ground that students trained in these grammars were quicker and keener in scientific observation. The psychological controversy about transfer of ability from one subject-matter to another always hangs on the discovery of common properties in the subject matters. It is not hard to find them in this case. As great an observer as Galileo spoke of his work in mechanics as decoding the book of nature, and he even gives us the middle language by which he made his translations, namely mathematics. The trick in finding the common ground for the book-worm grammarian and the observer of nature is not a difficult one. There is no more trickery in it than finding that Greek translates into English. It is only necessary to take stock of the languages one knows. There is the language in which we speak and write as members of the English culture group. There is also the language of an imagery in which we speak to ourselves and perhaps our families or best friends. There is the language of our gestures both conscious and unconscious. There is the language of our daily rituals such as washing, eating with knife and fork, wearing neckties and trousers or skirts ; by all these we say that we belong to European culture and believe its rules of prudence. But back of all these lies the non-artificial world of nature or as much of it as we are sensitive to, and all our languages, in so far as we are judged to be sane, bear an analogical correspondence to this basic language. If it were not for this so-called external world none of our notations would maintain their properties long enough for us to use them in communication. It is too often said that the ancient grammarians restricted their attention too much to the language of their books, but they would have the tu quoque answer that we restrict our attention too much to the language of the external world which humanly speaking is not as precise or elegant a language.

The ancient grammarian was concerned with the parts of speech and their relations in sentences from which he could extract significant patterns. The modern observer is concerned with the parts of the external world, their classification into mineral, vegetable, and animal, and their relations in experimental situations in which he can read significant patterns. He is the scientific grammarian. The experimental scientist and the engineer are the artist-grammarians who are writing their meanings in natural objects. It is important to realize that the world of empirical things, which for our ancestors was a medium for a practical art of life, is for us a natural notation, and that we in our modern science have become much more pedantic and scholarly about this natural notation than they thought of trying to be. It is the scientific pedant who insists on facts and their importance in science, and this is to praise him as we should praise the grammatical pedant of the Alexandrian period for the knowledge he gained from books and for the art of reading that he passed on to our tradition.

Much as the modern scientific observer dislikes to be classed with the grammarians, he would even more warmly renounce any claim to skill in rhetoric. It is a matter of conscience with him to leave other languages than his scientific language outside the laboratory door. But right there the trivial critic catches him smuggling in another language from his facts. He is at least engaged in correlating his scientific language with the natural language supplied by his facts. His monographs are translations of the facts into this scientific language, and in many cases the sheer bulk of such translation is the measure of his scientific capacity. His defence against this appearance of contamination from linguistic sources is that the scientific languages have come from the facts, and are therefore independently justified. So they are, but the techniques of justification are none the less parts of the ancient rhetorical art and extensions of it to new materials. It is of the nature of the rhetorical arts to expand and conquer just such new materials.

But there are still other languages which he will have no admitted part in, the language of the emotions, the language of trial and error operations, the language in which he has isolated and concealed his pre-conceived ideas. It is only necessary here to point out that his success in the laboratory is based on a training and skill which are finely mixed products of the emotional arts by virtue of which he prides himself on his coolness and impartiality, of the manual arts which he has practised from childhood up, and the cultural heritage which he could not escape. These are the stuff from which the originality of the genius, the laboratory atmosphere, and the international organization of science are made.

Finally the parallel parts played by authority in the ancient arts and scientific instruments in modern scientific techniques should cancel any accusations of bad faith levelled at those who can see ancient wisdom reincarnated in laboratory equipment. Ancient authorities dictated faith and practice ; so do instruments of precision. Ancient authorities laid down dogmas ; modern instruments set up standards. Ancient scholars compared and corrected authorities ; modern researchers compare and test their instruments. Ancient heresies were condemned for divergence from the established rules of procedure and new discovery of fact and idea were suspect until approved by official review ; modern research results must be reported in such terms that the experiment can be repeated with standard instruments. These are the correct social machinery for the advancement of any arts and sciences. Modern science has shed very little new light on the good and bad luck that attends those who preside over the assimilation of novelty to tradition.

The discovery of the lever and the wheel and the scientific development of their combinations have been the original revelation and the traditional growth of a faith which now operates not only in the mechanical, but also in the optical and electrical instruments of the modern laboratory and observatory. It is by the reading of instruments that the modern grammarian educes from himself and from things the laws and principles of nature. These final products are, of course, only the final sublimation of the grammars and rhetorics of science into the truths of science.

It is fashionable these days to use these terms, laws, principles, and truths, with modest qualification, as when we substitute for them hypotheses, assumptions, and correlations. This is because we have found that the liberal arts work fast in empirical material and yesterday's truths are to-day's discarded hypotheses. This caution and humility are to be found in the understatements and minor keys of the literary arts also. They are due to lack of insight into dialectical subtleties. In science when the formal insights fail, only facts are trusted. One simple statement should be enough to cure this failure of nerve : The liberal arts consist of formal operations performed on materials. The materials in the case of science are found in human experience, and they are capable of endless refinement by the successive applications of the liberal arts and sciences. Refinement depends on clarification, each operation achieving a degree of added clarity and providing a better ordered material for further clarification. Yesterday's discarded hypothesis yielded its measure of clarity and was on its own level of clarity a scientific truth, that is an abstract universal partially grasped in a notation. To-day's reformulation is another grasp of the same or related abstractions. To-morrow, with good luck and skill, it will yield a new formulation. It is only by the accumulation of facts that the abstraction appears to the intellect, but it is the abstractions in the intellect that remain to be further explored and further clarified.   The end result of science is clear abstractions, laws, principles, and truths in some notational mode which has been conditioned and qualified by notational accidents, instrumentation, axes of reference, available facts and human powers of observation and insight.   The history of science as of other modes of human thought does not show the coming-to-be and passing-away of truths, but rather the infinite grammatical modes in which truths can be discovered and formulated.   Degrees of clarity are relative to the historical patterns which these grammatical modes present.

There is implicit in this extension of the liberal arts an assumption that any concretely existent thing is potentially a symbol.   In other words, for the mind properly trained in the liberal arts any situation of immediately presented objects is a text to be read, rhetorically expanded, and logically interpreted.   This is a summary way, customary in the seventeenth century, of formulating the faith which since that time has been held by the natural scientist.   It says, on the one hand, that nature holds within its patterns certain discoverable uniformities. Further it says that things are governed by laws.   Finally it says that there are always empirical ways of discovering these uniformities and laws.   It is, of course, these ways that have been formalized and formulated in the trivium, but the tradition of which they are the medieval crystallization had a long history before the middle ages.   It is perhaps best expressed in the myth that now goes by the name, the doctrine of signatures.   This myth says that when God created man and made him subject to ills and misfortunes He also created stones, plants, animals, and other human beings and marked them with characteristic marks to be recognized and used as remedies. He gave man the ability to read these signatures both in himself and in natural objects and to interpret them for the good of his soul and body. Out of this medical Garden of Eden there have arisen the arts of life, in medicine the ancient arts of diagnosis, prognosis, and therapeutics ; in science the modern arts of observation, experimentation, and prediction ; in the life of the spirit the liberal arts, grammar, rhetoric, and logic. I have begun with the trivium because it presents the most general principles and the clearest distinctions. If I turn now to the medical arts and the natural sciences, it will be only to find these principles in more specific applications. It may serve the purposes of exposition better if I turn first to the natural sciences and examine the methods for reading the signatures in things. It may be interesting, by the way, to recall again the remark of Galileo that he was reading the book of nature by a decoding process that involved experimentation and measurement. Galileo began his higher education with medicine and then turned to physics—not an uncommon trope in the educational patterns of the time.

It would seem that there is a wide range of things that are obviously potential symbols or signatures. At one end of this range are the classical literary works of the past, which because of the intelligence and artistry of their authors are highly charged with symbolic significance. When we pay exclusive attention to the classics, we find a solid grammatical pattern in each work that carries precise meaning and rewards with ever deeper understanding, any amount of prolonged and detailed reading.   This means that good literature is rhetorically rich like a palimpsest in superimposed yet distinguishable layers of intellectual content.   The classics are like onions each of whose successive coverings contains complete onion essence.   Yet in spite of their final intelligibilities books taken as books are merely materials for the exercise of the liberal arts, reading, translating, etc.   They are as unintelligible as raw nature when they are taken as paper and ink.   This potentiality which they have may well be called in the medieval terms signate matter, matter which has on it the seal of the intellect.   Signate matter is realized in actual understanding by the art of observation.   Like nature literature begins as opaque fact and must be construed before it is read.

At the other end of the scale of potential symbols are apparent facts or natural phenomena.   These are also capable of being read, expanded, and logically interpreted. They are signate matter.   But the reading of natural phenomena leads to more subtle grammatical arts and newer grammatical distinctions than would be contained in the classical works on Grammar.   We shall need an art and a science of signatures.   Let us call an item of nature as observed in experience a signature.   This may be a crystal shape or the reading on the scale of an instrument. As in literary interpretation it will be assumed that the shape of the crystal or the number on the scale has a direct reference to something beyond itself, perhaps some other thing in the immediate situation.   It will have a first imposition. But in order to verify that imposition or reference it will be necessary to note the properties it has within its notational pattern. We must find its position and relations within the immediate context in order to fix its second imposition. In the case of words we must discover what part of speech a given unit is by noting the grammatical rules it obeys ; similarly in the case of a signature we must detect its functions in the phenomenal context. In ordinary scientific practice this is done by formulating a precise account of its space and time or space-time relationships with other designated items. As a matter of accuracy this involves noting many other features besides space-time relations, since the final space-time values are built on more elementary distinctions which are called for want of better names, qualitative. They go back ultimately to distinguishable items in crude unsophisticated experience and become steady and clear only by the application of what Kant called schemata, what we now call serial and structural patterns, or some more elaborate devices such as Mr. Whitehead's extensive abstraction. In spite of many brave philosophical attempts to study pure phenomenology of this kind, most of these patterns and devices still remain as rules of thumb and inarticulate habits. A great deal of linguistic grammar is in the same limbo, but we can see in scientific observation as well as in literature that we already have in our signatures the working of grammatical and rhetorical patterns by which a translation is made from qualitative differences to space and time relations. Observational data are construed in parallel series and the rhetorical leaps are made across the resulting analogy by insight and intuition into the common forms. The grammar of the signatures thus becomes clear and steady, and we can now recognize the proper second impositions, as we give the words the impositions of noun, verb, adjective, etc. In general, signatures in nature become observed properties and fall into regular patterns. In the more elaborate techniques of the modern laboratory this sort of thing is accomplished almost entirely in the setting up of the experimental situation, a process of juxta-position of instrument and material which imitates writing. Thus instruments are the automatic machines for determining the second impositions of signatures. They construe and parse the parts of the sentences and paragraphs in which nature speaks. They are reading machines, and their successful use in controlled observa-tion has cast considerable doubt on the efficiency and accuracy of the human reading machine in uncontrolled observation. The camera at the eye piece of a telescope has displaced the human eye so that now one wonders whether the human eye should be trusted even in reading the films that the camera prints. However, the final reading must be done by the human eye and reason, and if controls are still demanded, we have recourse to psychology and morals as final certificates of grammatical validity.

The determination of second impositions is, however, only preliminary and pre-requisite to the determination of first impositions. What does the observation " mean " ? As we have seen before there are two kinds of first imposition, concrete and abstract, and the preced-ing question is therefore ambiguous. It might better be put, What does the signature indicate? Concrete indications can be separated and treated discretely and thus the literal-minded confusion of a rhetorical manifold of references will be clarified and organized.

Suppose we take the number on a scale, or the form of a crystal. The number is a concrete number ; that is, it is not merely an arithmetic number, but a numbered somewhat, five pounds, ten feet, twenty volts. The geometric shape of the crystal is not merely a geometric figure, but a body in that shape. It is clear that they do not behave like pure mathematical entities when we try to apply mathematical operations to them. For instance, degrees of temperature cannot be multiplied according to the arithmetic rules for multiplication, and a very special branch of mathematics has to be invented *ad hoc* if we try to apply purely geometrical rules to the right- and left-handed figures of crystals. Concrete numbers are figures of speech, mathematical metaphors, and must be handled with rhetorical sophistication. Hence the theory of physical dimensions in physics, and the confusions in other sciences that are not provided with similar critical devices.

The trivial protection against this danger of confusion is the calculus or logic of analogies. A signature whose second impositions have been determined belongs to a notational expression which stands in analogy with some array of objects which have been construed in a similar grammatical pattern or schema. Thus the colours in the spectrum are ordered in a series and the formal order of that series is correlated or analogized with a set of numbers having a similar order. When we say red has a wavelength of 640, we are cutting across the analogy between

colours and numbers by a metaphorical route, talking at
least two languages of space and number with the sur-
reptitious introduction of a third language in which we
describe a disturbed pool of water. The calibrated
spectrometer has mechanically represented these three
languages and synthesized them, and we read off the
condensed result. It would be a mistake to try to add
the numbers that stand for wavelengths and hope to get
a result that would still be wavelengths; it might be still
more dangerous to train the objective of the spectrometer
on a smile illumined face and read off the vibration rate
of our sweetheart's personality. The mistakes would be
the same in principle. A great deal of the interdepart
mental talk between sciences and all work in applied
science   run   the   risk   of   being   Babelized   in   this
fashion.

The form of the analogy is important. As I have said
before, it provides a basis for the translation of the two
languages. The grammatical form of an observation may
be a spatial pattern within which the data appear on the
one hand, and a numerical pattern on the other. These
will be formally similar and therefore translatable, as the
numerical and qualitative languages of the spectrometer,
but this analogical scheme has more in it than immediately
meets the eye. The simple one-to-one correspondence of
colour and number is easy to read, but calculation of other
wavelengths by so-called interpolation or extrapolation
involves a network that may easily become tangled.
This danger makes scientists avoid the explicit use of
analogies, but they are repelled by fear rather than by
understanding.

The danger of entanglement arises from the following circumstance in the use of analogy. Take a simple four-termed analogy, A : B : : C : D. A and B connected by the sign of a ratio, : , are understood to be related in some grammatical fashion, either as words in a sentence, as points in space, as instants in time, or as cause and effect. The other ratio connects C and D in some similar way. Expressed verbally the formula says that there is at least one relation between A and B that is similar to at least one relation between C and D. It should be noted that in spite of the indefiniteness of the ratio with respect to specific relations, we can still maintain the analogy and for purposes of calculation assume that A and C are connected by what I shall call a line of signification ; A signifies C by virtue of their corresponding positions in similar ratios. In the same way B signifies D. But if the analogy is well built, we can take the analogy by alternation thus A : C : : B : D, and this means that there is at least one relation between A and C that is similar to at least one relation between B and D. Then as before A will signify B and C will signify D by virtue of their respective corresponding positions in similar ratios. The reader will appreciate from the difficulty of following this exposition why the scientist fears analogies, why the poet revels in them, and, therefore, why it is important that someone, a master of the arts, should make it his business to analyse them. The analysis follows the model that Euclid lays down in his treatment of numerical and geometrical proportions. Alternation is one of his transformations and in it, as applied above, one can see the necessity of maintaining the distinction between grammatical relations and lines of signification. This diagram may help to present the two cases and the detail of the transformation.

$$
\begin{array}{ccccc}
A : B & & A \rightarrow B & & A : C \\
\downarrow \ \downarrow & & \cdot\cdot \ \ \cdot\cdot & \text{or} & \downarrow \ \downarrow \\
C : D & & C \rightarrow D & & B : D
\end{array}
$$

The analogy thus understood provides the context for the distinctions between terms in first and second impositions. Each term in the above formulae is taken in both impositions ; A is in second imposition when its context is its ratio, A : B ; A is taken in first imposition when its context is the whole analogy and it signifies C. But alternation reverses the impositions so that A is taken in second imposition in the ratio A : C, and in a corresponding first imposition as signifying B. It is fairly obvious, though not always recognized, that artificial symbols such as words may have these complicated modes of signifying ; it is not so obvious, and it is a bit disturbing, to realize that natural things as soon as they come within the experience of the observer, have equally if not more complicated modes of signifying. It is perhaps even more disturbing that the extension of the liberal arts into the natural world has brought with it the intellectual obligation to be as subtly artistic in science as poets and literary critics have been in literature. We are constantly faced with problems that require this subtlety for their solution when we try to interpret observation and measurement. The instruments supply us with signatures in patterns. With sufficient ingenuity their second impositions, that is their grammatical relations, can be divined and formulated. This means that we get one side of an analogy, and lines of signification stretch out like tentacles seeking the termini of the first impositions. When these are discovered either by more observation or by imaginative construction, as in the making of hypotheses, they turn out to be more signatures in grammatical patterns. We should recognize the analogical structure at that point and note the lines of signification that connect the corresponding terms of the two analogues. But instead of that we immediately jump to the transformation of the analogy by alternation and substitute some grammatical relation for the lines of signification. By taking only the grammatical relations from the two forms of the analogy and putting them together in one pattern we arrive at a third grammatical pattern containing four terms thus: A : B : C : D. This then becomes one side of a more complex analogy and we hunt again for the lines of signification that will lead to the other side. We may follow the same procedure with this analogy and end up again without an answer to the question, What do signatures indicate? This procedure results in the collection of many patterns and uniformities. Its success persuades philosophers that it is the whole of scientific method, and their statement of it has been made into the positivistic and phenomenalistic doctrines under which we still work. These doctrines amount to the denial that any lines of signification exist, although these lines have been the guiding threads of the procedure which they describe.

All this belongs to the rhetoric of science and has had in the course of its history many clever turns of imagination and reasoning. The medievals, having watched these turns with subtle attention, summarized their conclusions in the doctrine that lines of signification were the inverse of lines of causation so that an effect was a sign of its cause. We follow the same doctrine when we say that smoke is a sign of fire. If X is the cause of Y, then Y is the sign of X. By this they did not mean the causal relation is the same as a line of signification ; the fact that one is the inverse of the other may, and usually does, mean that they are quite different, though the two meanings are connected with each other as we have found them in the analogy taken by alternation. Causation is symbolized in the grammatical notational relation in each side of the analogy, but the terms of this relation may also be related otherwise by lines of signification. Briefly, two things may be connected in two different ways, in one way by causal efficacy or space-time juxtaposition, and in the other through a different analogical context by lines of signification. Identification of the two ways would be confusing very different relations. These two ways of relating terms have been distinguished by Professor Whitehead in his *Symbolism : Its Meaning and Effects.* He speaks there of two modes of symbols, one by causal efficacy, the other by presentational immediacy. He is interested in the special case of signs as they function in perception, where objects causally effect sensations, and also become objects of reflective consciousness. In the analogy this distinction is generalized and shows how the two may be confused, not only in perception, but in all cases of things in relation signifying other things in similar relations.

We can now give a part of the answer to the question, What do signatures signify ? The signate matter of observation, the pattern of observed data, forms one side of an analogy. It signifies the other side of that analogy. The other side of the analogy (and there may be several analogues, as in the case of numbers, colours, and ether waves) might ideally be another clear pattern of observed data. If the scientist were concerned merely with the explanation of man-made machines, this would be the case. The external appearance and performance of the machine would supply his observed material, one side of the analogy. He could then take the machine to pieces and find the internal parts and their articulations, and these would constitute a pattern grammatically similar to the external pattern. To a certain extent this is possible with natural objects, not man-made. Early modern science was very successful with this sort of pattern making and correlating of internal and external parts. But even here difficulties arose which became insurmountable with more delicate or invisible parts, and constructive imagination had to step in as an artificial aid. Mechanical models of the molecule were imagined and sometimes constructed to scale where the actual object under investigation would not allow further division, or where the microscope blurred instead of magnifying. The indivisible and the invisible borrowed their parts from imagination and Euclidean geometry. When these failed, operational mathematics became the inventor of sub-microscopic machines and tiny demonic demiurges were set to tend flocks of wayward molecules. Mathematics and mechanical imagination work together with the pre-established harmony that binds infinitesimals together to provide unseen analogues for the observed signatures, and we have Newtonian physics and astronomy, Daltonian chemistry, and undulatory thermodynamics and electrodynamics. These support the moral confidence with which scientists from the seventeenth to the nineteenth century answer the question of significance : Signatures signify machines—or atoms.

But this proved to be only the beginning of the romantic period in modern science. The betrothal of imagination and mathematics soon proved fruitful of other than mechanical analogues with which observed phenomena could be correlated and measured. Rays, particles, and waves were collected and recollected from experience, and the newer mathematical devices arising from newer symbolic devices in pure mathematics have brought us to our modern astrophysical and subatomic cosmological patterns and maps. God has been good to us in marking the remedies of our discontents with visible signs, but He has gone farther in His mercy in giving us mathematics and imagination by which we can invent signatures where there are no things to see. These are the end terms of the first impositions that we put on the signatures which we have isolated in experience by the techniques of observation.

In the course of discussing observation I have had little occasion to mention techniques, instruments, and operations. Of course what I said pre-supposed a great deal of technology. No direct attention has been paid to this aspect so far because if it had been attended to we should have been obliged to keep too many themes going at once. Perhaps that is the reason that talk about scientific method in general has ignored technology until very recently.

What I have discussed is that aspect of science which parallels or extends the arts of reading and interpretation where operations and technique are subtle and difficult to catch on the wing. Nevertheless they have been present and it is now time to turn to that aspect of science that is called experimentation. Strictly speaking observation and experimentation are not separable, for in every observation there is a component of control, at least of attention, and every experiment is performed for what it will provide in the way of observable data.

Operations are the elementary units of control. They are of various sorts, ranging from the almost unnoticed changes in observation by a shift of attention to gross manipulations of materials by hand or by power. Mathematicians perform operations by shifting marks on paper and engineers perform operations with steam shovels and electric cranes. Grammarians and logicians proper perform operations by following a train of imagery in their mind's eye or by formulating an oral or written argument. Operations are performed whenever something is changed into something else according to a rule implicit or explicit. Operations are motions.

One of the great difficulties in treating them explicitly is their evanescence. It may be admitted that marks on paper express ideas, but it is only in gesture language that it is obvious that the motions of things express ideas. Consequently it is a late stage in science in which the scientist becomes critically aware of operations. In fact it has been the difficulties in mechanical and other imaginary and mathematical models that have brought operations to the foreground. When the models seemed

inadequate or inconsistent, as in the case of the lumini-
ferous ether, the mathematical physicist began answering
the problem of signification by saying that the signatures
were values in mathematical equations. Asked by the
experimental physicist what the equations signified he
flatteringly answered that they signified operations with
instruments. Equations are the rules for the operations
which are to be performed with instruments. The
experimental physicist was for the moment pleased that
his operations were the beginning and the end of physics,
but then noted that he was performing experimental
operations for the sake of discovering the rules of these
operations; the lines of significance had again disappeared. The philosopher finds the paradox illuminating, not merely because he has caught the physicist in a
typical squirrel cage, but because of the light that it
throws on the nature of operations.

The secret that the operation conceals is found in
certain symbolic properties it has in addition to the
dynamic properties of causing change in materials.
Operations like words and gestures refer beyond themselves not merely to things but also to ideas by lines of
signification to be recognized as second intentions. This
is concealed as well as suggested when it is said that
operations accord with rules; for rules on examination
turn out to be general propositions referring to any case
of a given kind, and their first intentions are usually
directed to future situations, that is situations that are
not yet actual. They are predictions, and they are
fulfilled and tested by operations. It is thus through
predictions and operations that experimental controls

enter the technique or art of the practising scientist. The science corresponding to this art or technique is expressed in the laws of nature which the operations obey.

Manual and instrumental operations introduce another grammatical pattern into the set of analogies that constitute the experimental situation, or another ratio into the process of measurement. In this grammatical pattern, ratio, or analogue, the things operated upon have taken the places of signatures of observation and the operations have taken the places of the relations. This new ratio or analogue can be taken as basic to the others which then become the termini of its lines of signification, or if the lines of signification are ignored the experimental series of operations can be made to carry the whole burden of significance. Eddington's pointer readings and instrument settings play this sort of role. But when this is the interpretation something like the catastrophe in tragedy takes place in the dramas of experimentation. Operations come and go, and the observer is left staring at nothing, and this evanescent character of observations subjected to operational analysis, turns the attention of the observer, who is the hero of the drama, to the laws that are not merely of to-day or of yesterday. If he has insight, his intellect grasps universals and isolates them from the flux. Empirical science suffers a sublimation, and the common form of the analogues begs for a reformulation independent of its more particular embodiments.

The importance of experimentation in science is largely due to the fact that it forces this sublimation ; it is disciplinary. In order to perform a truly experimental operation the experimenter must at some point in the process have abstract ideas to act as guiding principles. Otherwise he will not be able to set up apparatus that will make relevant and precise observation and measurement possible. The apparatus must be understood to embody accurately some principle or set of principles. Experimentation then forces a double clarification, first, the formulation of an abstract principle and, second, the exemplification of it in as single and exclusive a medium as can be found or made. Of course there are merely trial and error procedures in the laboratory, proper to the exploratory stages in an investigation when the use of analogies is the dominant procedure, but sharp clarity and precise embodiment must replace these first approximative procedures. Hence that super-technology, the making of instruments of precision. What is left over as necessary error must be held in check by singleness of mind and the direction of attention on the principles that lie back of the instrument.

Precision demands a sharp line to divide experimental materials into two classes, first, the controlled material which is directly submitted to experimental operations, and, second, the " controls " which are excluded from the experimental situation for the purpose of comparing and checking the procedure and bringing only relevant things to light. The original aim of experiment may have been to discover a new way to control nature, but the immediate aim must be the isolation of the material so that it may faithfully reveal its principles.

The usual aim assigned by philosophers to the processes of experimentation is the verification of hypotheses, and this is said either to establish a hypothesis as a law or to increase its probability by the adduction of evidence. Neither of these aims is practicable if their concealed intention is to provide proof. Both processes contain formal fallacies. But if establishing an hypothesis or increasing its probability means the improvement of its manifest embodiment and the consequent clarification of its meaning, then the process of verification belongs to the trivial arts, to that part of rhetoric which traces the bonds betwen the logic and the grammar of the experimental situation by translating abstraction into concrete terms—in other words, the rendering of an obscure subject matter intelligible by the arts of grammar and logic. Precision in instrumental operations and logical formulation appears in this context as the transforming of loose analogies into sets of compendent and rigorous propositions, and this is accomplished by the substitution of explicit determinate relations for the indefinite implicit ratios of the analogy. When the relations have been fixed in this way, the ratios turn into explicit propositions which can be distributed to their proper categories and arranged in deductive systems as constituting rational sciences.

The remaining part of the answer to the question, What do signatures signify ? is contained in this account of experimentation, prediction, and verification. The previous answer was that signatures in grammatical patterns signify other signatures in analogous patterns. The present answer adds second intentions. Signatures in grammatical patterns taken together in analogical correlations signify abstract ideas, the laws that science seeks. Correlation of signatures leads to the sublimation of scientific data and the abstraction of systems of ideas. The insight which follows the lines of signification finally focuses on forms that can then be reformulated in technical and precise language.

When the abstractions are finally grasped, the new terms in the general propositions will have first intentions as well as second intentions. The termini of these first intentions will be the observed data, signate matter, which when thus rationally ordered become facts. Signatures are thus transformed from things signifying to things signified by the new abstract formulae, and they are solid intelligible facts only in this context. If they are not fortunate enough to gain such articulation in general propositions, they are illusory appearances, wandering images, certainly enough observed and marked as signatures, but very uncertainly held in scientific repute, awaiting a happier adventure in the arts.

CHAPTER III

IN this exposition of the ways of the liberal arts with scientific material I have borrowed the term " signature " from the history of medicine. I have done this for several reasons. One is that its immediate connotation suggests the complicated ambiguities of the observed data in science. " Signate matter " makes a similar point, namely that the data in empirical science are unordered materials, but at the same time they have enough determinate form to seek and seize upon the intellectual orders proper to them. The first level of scientific fact presents a wavering flickering phosphorescent intellectual light. Scientific findings certainly have meaning, but we do not know just what they mean. Secondly, the term signature and the myth within which it occurs serves as a reminder of the historical roots of the natural sciences in medicine. One after another the seeds of the natural sciences have been blown by the winds of philosophical doctrine from the ancestral soil of the medical faculty of the medieval university and have taken independent roots in alien soil which has been cultivated by separate laboratories. Many of our verbal usages celebrate the ancient ancestry ; for instance, modern " physics " has only specialized " physic ", the former name of medicine. But there is more than verbal usage to signalize the derivation. The physician still passes his unsolved problems to the physicist, and waits for a filial answer, and the physicist continually pays his debt of piety by replying in refined terminology and an almost too ingenious technology. The doctor's office, perhaps too ostentatiously, exhibits the evidence of the physicist's helping hand in the array of physical instruments. So it is also with the chemist, botanist, and zoologist, though they are often ashamed of old-fashioned impurities that medical practice introduces into their scientific purity. It might perhaps be wise to allow the payment of the debt to be made through the philosophical clearing-house ; the philosophical transactions so introduced might lead to the discovery of a more workable medium of intellectual and practical communication and eliminate the confusions that now bring quackery into medicine and metaphysical nostalgia to the scientist. Even the laboratory technician might understand his work in a more humane context if he recalled his prototype in the practising physician and consequently recognized the manifold incidences of his art on human work and thought. At any rate " signature " is one of those never quite forgotten traditional terms to which we may have recourse when we wish to discover the genesis of natural science from medicine or when we face the practical problem of making science more effective in contemporary medicine.

If we think of the data of scientific observation as material in various degrees of elaboration, we can correlate the prejudices of the specialists in a given science with these degrees. The mathematical physicist will have nothing to do with the engineer's crudities because he has practised a very special art on high grade signatures. The engineer, on the other hand, will bridle at the niceties of the laboratory because his materials are much nearer to a primitive state of nature where significances are organized for a different purpose and accidents are allowed for rather than controlled. The laboratory physicist in his turn will wink at the vagaries of the mathematician and patronize the engineer because neither of them are single-minded in their respect for the instrument. The medical man, whether he works in the laboratory, the clinic, or in general practice, has to take account of signatures in all states of refinement, and furthermore, he has to take them from whatever source they are available, work them over, combine and separate them, and finally recombine them as signs not only of the operation of general laws, but also of the immediately present state of an individual organism. Hence his arts will be different : diagnosis, prognosis, and therapeutics instead of observation, prediction, and experimentation.

There is often confusion about the aims and achievements of the physician, and the physicist, and it is usually expressed in the question whether the physician is an artist or a scientist. It is said on the one side that the physician is always faced with a practical emergency, and even in the laboratory, the urgency and complexity of the vital process does not allow time or opportunity for trial and error, the testing of multiple working hypotheses, measurement, and successive verifications with the averaging of probable errors. The physician's work is therefore merely an art which at best can be respectable only in empirical practical ways. On the other side, it is less often said that the ways of the laboratory are merely manipulatory and imaginative arts which with their greatest refinements only reach probabilities and approximations.   The more rigorous the intellectual processes that are brought to bear on laboratory problems, the more obvious it becomes that the results are opinions, with more or less elaborate non-intellectual justifications.   Thus both physician and physicist turn out to be artists.   A similar pair of arguments can be arrayed to show that both are scientists.   For the physician can show that he never is allowed to stop with an apology for his opinion ; he must sharply separate what he opines from what he knows, and by professional mandate act on only what he knows. This emphasis on genuine knowledge is recorded in the terms diagnosis and prognosis, where the ending *gnosis* connotes substantial knowledge.   On the other hand, the knowledge of the physician is only partly made up of the understanding of general laws which are the proper subject matter of science in the strict sense.   The physician must understand the general laws, but he must also know that the individual before him is a genuine case of these laws.   The physicist, on the other hand, can avoid this demand by collecting many possible cases and calculating the probability of the general law operating in similar material.

One can see here there is cause enough for confusion and reason to suspect that art and science are too closely associated in both physics and medicine to allow for an easy analysis and separation.   Certainly the simple faith that progress in the natural sciences has made, or will make, direct contributions to the medical arts cannot hope to establish itself on the conventional supposition that science is made only in the laboratory and cures are made only at the bedside.

When an "interesting" patient is brought to the hospital and emergency measures have been taken to meet the acute symptoms that have occasioned hospitalization, the person becomes the object of attention from one physician directly and indirectly or potentially from the whole staff of the institution, and his welfare becomes the end for the sake of which the entire institutional equipment may be set in motion. Let us say that the acute symptoms have proved amenable to the emergency measures, and therefore that diagnosis, prognosis, and therapy have already taken their first steps, perhaps in a very short space of time, and so mutually implicated that it is difficult to formulate them separately even for the purposes of description. An acute symptom was noted, a remedy popped into the mind of the physician at the same time with his recognition of the symptom and an inference of its probable cause and consequences, the remedy was immediately administered and its effects noted. We already have a very complicated mixture of art and science in the case record. The symptom or complex of symptoms classified the patient in the physician's mind, and the context of possible causes, consequences, and remedies were perhaps memorized deductions from a well-known medical theory, selected on the basis of medical experience with similar symptoms, and modified to fit the constitutional type and peculiar characteristics of the patient.

The prognostic phase of the judgment is hardly to be

distinguished in this context, but we can see that it was present in the inference that was at least implicitly made in the selection of therapeutic measures. The remedy was given in order to change the symptom which would have continued or got worse. This inference depends on a dilemma between a prediction of the course of the trouble if left alone, and a prediction of the effect of the remedy if it is administered. The effect when it occurred was a further diagnostic finding verifying within the limits of the situation the previous diagnosis and its prognostic and therapeutic implications. It is important to note the ambivalence of the data as they fall into their first rubrics. Diagnosis is the primary basis for the prognosis and the therapy, prognosis revises the primary diagnosis and suggests other symptoms to be looked for in a therapeutic context. Therapy always uncovers more diagnostic symptoms and prognostic possibilities and removes some of the original symptoms. It would be possible to describe the whole situation and development as any one of the three arts with the other two as merely subsidiary parts. All of them together place the patient in the framework of professional knowledge which the physician embodies in the three artistic phases.

When the patient in the ideal case has been allowed to adjust himself to hospital routine, the systematic attention given him follows a more extended elaborate dramatic pattern with the three medical arts playing similarly interrelated but more discernible roles. His regimen, which includes not only what he eats and drinks, but also how much and what kind of rest and activity he is allowed, as well as the control of the more intangible parts of his environment, is devised not only to bring about his ease and recovery, but also by establishing known conditions to uncover still hidden symptoms that may be relevant. Hospitals, at first under the auspices of monasteries and therefore under strict standardized controls, are the cultural ancestors of the laboratory where cases are isolated and watched under constant conditions. It is only thus that nature shows her signatures. The hospital bed is perhaps the standard plane which Galileo inclined in order to read the signatures of falling bodies.

The inveterate antipathy and fear of the hospital that the potential patients and their relatives show is partly due, of course, to the natural repugnance to serious illness and death, but it is also due in part to the sublimation that the patient undergoes. He loses his individuality as soon as he is assigned to a physician and a ward, and his adjustment to the new world is an initiation into a society which proceeds to label its members with abstract and esoteric terms, names that the medical arts confer upon their subjects as irrevocably as the cattle-puncher with his branding iron. These names are the products of the diagnostic and therapeutic arts, certified signatures that fix a status, promise a future, and define services due the person.

Perhaps it would be less disturbing to say that the patient has become a personae dramatis with an assigned role in a miracle or morality play. The action that ensues has a realistic appearance but the issues and conflicts are more concerned with the abstractions of science than with the individual motives and values of the actor.

It is important to keep this ritualistic and impersonal aspect of medicine in mind and to recognize in it one of the most impressive survivals of the old medical tradition that helps to make modern scientific techniques effective in medicine.   It is even more important to remember this when one is noting the simulation of personal regard that goes by the name of bedside manner.   Perhaps there is no professional code that manages to maintain so much of the normal and familiar human relationships as the medical code.   But this should not obscure the double entendre of medical manners.   A great deal of the professional medical code is only a formalization of good social manners for laboratory purposes.

It is into this highly formalized context that the details of the patient's biography are introduced.   Age, sex, occupation, marital state, and the manner in which the patient has met past physical, social, and spiritual crises come under diagnostic scrutiny.   It is only the physician's capacity to see the abstract in the concrete that limits the relevance of such details, and a case record should contain at least as much information as the hospital staff as a group can assimilate to the professional code.   In practice of course the amount of such details and the relative weight they carry will presumably be determined by many accidental features of the situation, and perhaps the fashions and moods that happen to influence the diagnostician.   At present, for instance, it is fashionable in the medical wards to slur over so-called neurotic symptoms and purposely to underestimate events with which they are connected, partly because the therapy for neurosis seems uncertain and partly because the medical man hopes to reduce many neurotic symptoms to their physical correlates.

As the case history is being acquired gross observation of surface symptoms continues, items of history and items of observation combining to determine lines of inquiry. These lines of inquiry may in turn lead to palpation, percussion, auscultation, and the whole array of instrumental techniques that are interpretable through one or another special science or some combination that they dictate. These range from the gross observation of pallor or cyanosis to the determination of the state of the retina with the ophthalmoscope, or other hidden conditions with the thermometer, the stethoscope, and the rubber mallet. It will be noted that some of these observations end in judgments of greater or less than the norm, and that some of them give precise judgments of degree based on calibrations in the instruments. It is with subtleties like this that the lines of inquiry run through series of tests where the notion of a norm merely represents a base line by reference to which graded judgments of more or less can be made. Diagnosis is here getting into deep waters and taking on a mysterious aspect if it faces the theoretical questions. Such questions are very complex. If a norm is taken to be the state of health or safety of a given part, the well-trained physician will recall the wide range of possible safe variation in the healthy states of single organs in various individuals, and he will probably retreat to the notion of variable norms. The variations in individuals are so great that unless the patient under consideration has been an invalid under regular and prolonged medical treatment, his individual norm cannot be known.   Norms vary from day to day in supposedly healthy persons enough to upset most workable standards. Statistical techniques have been borrowed from special fields of science to justify the assumption of norms that will be mean values between extremes of variation, but if we follow this we are in the field of insurance or group physiology and have left any contemporary hospital practice.   In view of all this it seems best to assume that diagnostic norms are merely arbitrary zero points for making descriptive and relative judgments for standard records.

Laboratory tests are made while the gross physical observations are supplying data for the superficial symptom pattern.   A superficial symptom or a crisis in the history suggests associated internal states, and the relevant series of tests is ordered.   Specimens of urine, faeces, sputum, blood, gastro-intestinal contents, or spinal fluid are taken to the laboratory.   The traditional tests or their latest chemical and physical refinements are applied and the results are incorporated in the record. The fashion here is to put these results in numerical terms even when concrete numbers have not been put through a critical ordering such as that called dimensions in physics.   The laboratory does not judge divergence from the norm, but merely gives the descriptive numerical values and leaves the strictly medical judgment to the physician.

If surgery has intervened there may be sections of tissues or whole organs removed for pathological analysis, and this may lead to another round of laboratory tests, by cytologists, biochemists, and biophysicists.   Any of the above specimens or sections may also be sent to the bacteriologist, and the whole technique of preparing and testing cultures may be brought into operation.   Finally X-ray photographs may ,be taken and read, or the psychiatrist may be called in for review and consultation. Some psychiatrists at present wish they had as imposing a piece of apparatus as the X-ray camera to add prestige to their judgments—a wish that shows the present preponderance of prestige in favour of the physical laboratories.

Let us suppose now for purposes of description that the lines of inquiry have been transformed into series of findings and that history, superficial observation, and fine analysis have been completed and condensed into a table of findings.   Up to this point there has been no genuine diagnostic judgment. Anything approaching such a judgment has been tentative and heuristic in its intention ; one finding has led to another finding by the routes of regimen and therapy or by the less tangible ways of the trained imagination and intellect of the diagnostician.   If the story were told in terms of contemporary theory of science and scientific method, the process would be called observation, controlled observation, hypothesis-making, experimentation and verification.   Perhaps a more accurate description would come from the man of common-sense, who would talk about looking, listening, prodding, getting a hunch, and taking notes.   Both of these would leave out the parts of the process that make medicine a profession.   In the back of the physician's mind, though seldom made explicit enough to be caught and put down in a manual, there are formal schemes of categories, genera, and species, across and up-and-down which his mind moves. These may be abstract universals, but more likely as generic images, since the universals appear in the mind clothed in imagery which has accumulated from the physician's experience. The memory of a previously observed symptom provides such an image-concept and it may belong with other similar or related images in an apperceptive mass. These imaginative patterns are continually growing and changing as diagnosis proceeds but always according to laws of association which on analysis turn out to be rules of logic, rules for the subsumption of concepts or classes. Logical opposites may turn out to be contradictories and in time will be dissociated, or they may turn out to be contrary co-ordinate species under a common genus, or subsumed one under the other in a genus-species hierarchy. A symptom recognized is an infima species under a hierarchy of species which is topped by a summum genus. The symptom itself is ambiguous because it can and usually does belong to more than one such hierarchy. It suggests many lines of inquiry running up these hierarchies, across and down to other infimae species which may be looked for in the case. Suggestion and explorative inferences, if made explicit, would fall into dilemmas, hypothetical propositions and syllogisms, and the other devices of formal logic by which the mind moves in many directions among its objects. Since these suggestions and inferences seldom are explicit, the process seems one-dimensional, obscure, lightning-like, and personal, even to the extreme of being subconscious. The superficial appearance of the diagnostic process is a good deal like painting, a stroke here, a stroke there, and perhaps at the end the picture jumps from the canvas to the eye, or perhaps it doesn't.   Actually the eye and the mind of the painter have been behind the strokes, and likewise the eye and the mind of the observer are involved in the observation, so that when the strokes are right with respect to the eye and the mind, the picture is created.   But the operation of the eye and the mind do not directly exhibit the species-genus hierarchy of formal logic.   Fortunately the similarities and differences of the materials spontaneously fall into analogical patterns that easily and speedily imitate formal logic, and the secret of the painter and the physician lies in their skill in detecting the logic implicit in analogies.   Analogical insights tend to move across rather than up and down the hierarchy, and they thus allow the observer to keep close to the concrete materials, the pigments, or the symptoms.

   The diagnostic conclusion leaps to the eye perhaps early in the investigation of the case, but it leaps because the mind has prepared a place for it to land, and a good mind can always find more than one such place.   A good diagnosis of an interesting case is always the dialectical statement of several possibilities.   The answer to the question, What is wrong with the patient, is always analysable into a set of alternatives, or a system of dilemmas.   This is so even though there may be a simple pathological name for the disease or diseases present. The reason for this apparently evasive answer is very simple, but the route to it is beset by many subtleties, and the consequences are often upsetting both to the medical man and the layman who is a potential patient.

   It will be recalled that the patient on entering the

hospital lost his individuality to a degree and achieved a status and a role in this new isolated world of abstract scientific standards. This initiation may appear to have happened suddenly and completely on admission, but actually the recognition of the first symptom was merely the first stage in a process that has been continuing throughout the diagnostic investigation and its borrowings from prognosis and therapy. Each recognized and recorded item of the case history has uncovered some further characteristic of the patient and placed a corresponding abstraction in relation to others like it. At the same time the institution has set the relevant parts of its equipment into operation, and the corresponding abstractions, like pieces of equipment, have affinities. As one test leads to another, so one abstracted symptom leads to another. The physician's mind may have jumped ahead of the process and seen the final judgment coming, but the actual judgment is not made until the hospitalization has completed the course of its operations, and the abstractions have built a system. In a scientific laboratory this would be called a theory, and would be stated as a hypothetical proposition, if such and such, then so and so. The prognostic statement is something like that but in diagnosis the dilemmatic statement of alternatives is the rule. The reason for this is that the patient as an individual must not be lost sight of in the application of the medical sciences. He is the many-sided subject of the diagnostic judgment. A simple judgment could only indicate that he is sick, but that would not be an illuminating medical statement. The related alternative predicates substituted for " sick ", mark the presence of scientific abstractions. It would seem that " John has typhoid fever " would be a simple scientific statement, but it really is no better than " John is sick ", except for the lay person. The scientific statement is a very complicated array of predicates connected by various logical relations that are best expressed in alternative predicates of a singular subject, the patient as individual. The preliminary diagnostic trial judgments have been made in a tentative mood and their proper form has been hypothetical. They have been dealing with universals only, but the genuine, though perhaps not final diagnostic judgment has the complex individual as its subject, and the single simple predicate that we as human beings seek must be made explicit in the set of alternatives and perhaps has no integrated name at all. It would add very little to the alternatives to give them such a name ; it would be like adding the term dormitive powers to explain the sleep that morphine brings.

It is true that medical men make other points when they talk about this peculiarity of diagnostic judgments. They are apt to confuse the tentative explorative judgments with the diagnosis proper, and pride themselves on their final open-mindedness, and their philosophical scepticism ; or they may stress the purely pragmatic incidence of diagnosis, thus emphasizing unduly the connection that diagnosis has with therapy ; or they may emphasize the limitations of medical knowledge and thus play up the moral heroism of the medical profession facing life and death with Quixotic boldness. On the other hand, the frightened or disdainful lay person may contract a disgust for such wishy-washy professional indecision, and look for the quack who just cures sick people without claptrap. All these are mistaking the rigour and explicitness of *either* . . . *or* propositions with their vulgar use to express degrees of ignorance of indecision. One may explain the physicist's meaning for " colour " by saying either red, yellow, green, or blue or violet ; or the lady customer at the ribbon counter may ask whether red, or yellow, or purple will go with red hair.

The " either—or " form of the diagnostic judgment is the technical way a physician has of stating what medical science finds out about a patient, just as the equally puzzling algebraic equation is the way a physicist has of stating what he has found out about falling bodies. The equation could be stated as a complicated set of alternatives ; and the diagnostic judgment could be stated in good mathematical form if the physician knew a very small minimum about the techniques of mathematical logic. This leaves out the fundamental difference between the intent of the physician and that of the physicist. The physicist wants the statement of a general law, the physician the analytic statement of the condition of an individual.

With regard to the last question it is sometimes said hat the reason for the apparent tentative status of the diagnostic judgment is the incompleteness of information, the relative impossibility of seeing the inside of living bodies, or of catching the passing symptom on the wing. These are ironies that haunt all scientific inquiry and there is much difficulty in keeping them within rational bounds. Frightened by a necessary relative incompleteness in theory there are some medical men who look for an empirical completion by the autopsy room.   There is a narrow door which all have to pass, and where the social difficulties are at a minimum.   Let the pathologist look at the real trouble there and fix the diagnosis and eliminate the medical man's guesses.   The trouble with this is that the autopsy room adds only more symptoms from another art, pathological anatomy, and that, in spite of their apparent strategic importance, they are neither clearer in significance, nor are they any more conclusive as evidence than any other fragmentary parts of the picture.   In short, they are to be assimilated in the same fashion as the data from the X-ray machine.   Temporal finality which seems to hang about the autopsy room is not to be identified with theoretical finality.   This is but one of a thousand fallacies that dogmatic empiricism has brought with it and has to keep with it in order to maintain its exclusive position of authority in contemporary science.

The status of time in all scientific investigation, or if you like in nature, is brought to view very vividly and typically in the art of prognosis.   Perhaps the most important distinction and relation between diagnosis and prognosis is to be made in terms of time.   Diagnosis detemporalizes the disease process, and prognosis unrolls even a momentary state into a significant time sequence. It was remarked above how quickly and apparently automatically the recognition of the acute symptom of the interesting patient passed over into an inference about the consequences of leaving it alone or applying a remedy. It seems as if the recognition were in itself a prophecy, and that is in fact the case.   Their separate formulations are two analyses of a single insight, one concerned with patterns and the other with processes, the single insight having as its actual object something that is both pattern and process.   It is plausible to assume that the morphological and the genetic themes in modern science took their origins in these two medical arts ; Professor Whitehead's metaphysics is founded on the identity of the objects or events that have these two analyses.

However sharply they may be distinguished in starting points, terminology, and results, it is not easy to disentangle them as they occur in hospitals.   The practising physician would say that there is a great deal of prognosis in diagnosis and a great deal of diagnosis in prognosis, and let it go at that.   This is so true superficially that it almost obscures the genuine distinction.   It may be possible to keep the distinction and yet see the interweaving relations if we say that for every diagnostic conclusion there is a genetic story.   Prognosis constructs stories with beginnings, middles, and ends.   The medical man has to begin in *medias res*, working both backwards and forwards to make the history as nearly a biography as possible.

In the account of diagnosis I have stressed the implicit logical pattern that becomes explicit as the picture is filled in.   In prognosis the underlying pattern is temporal instead of logical, but, as any story teller knows, temporal order alone does not constitute narrative or genetic form. In science there have been attempts to reduce causal series to the temporal series, but even in the most successful attempts there is always the smuggling in of some non-temporal principle.   The first notations in a medical case seem to approach the purely temporal ordering of symptoms and processes, and during the explorative stages the physician is very careful not to import any question-begging causal principles, but in spite of scruples there is more than precedence and succession in the unavoidable assumption that symptoms develop. Hence since there is no valid causal interpretation to be found in the mere order of discovery of the symptoms, each symptom is taken as representing the present stage of some process, earlier stages of which may be found if one looks to causal as well as chronological principles.

It is important for the full development of the story itself that each of the leading symptoms and their supposed geneses be kept separate and traced independently. Otherwise the plots will fuse and obscure the process. It is also important that no single plot shall dominate the early investigation and eclipse others. The biography is therefore allowed to split up into independent plots, each attaching itself as a line of inquiry to an outstanding diagnostic theme. Thus a number of corresponding time series are set up imaginatively to distinguish groups of symptoms and to put them in their proper genetic order, and these are allowed to extend into the future as routes along which new symptoms are to be sighted and picked up as the case progresses. The success of both these explorative procedures, causal and chronological, will depend upon the physician's knowledge of previous cases and his ability to vary the traditional patterns to fit the actual array of data.

It is not long in the watching of a case before time comes in not only as the serial order in which observed data can be placed, but also in such a way that temporal patterns themselves become data. It was a great day for both physics and medicine when Galileo compared two periodic rhythms, that of the pendulum and that of his pulse, and standardized them for science in general. So one may note periodic time patterns in pulse and breathing rates, and then build up periods in the rates of change of these rates. It may seem perverse to call this sort of thing prognosis, but it is a classical case of an inter-relation of diagnosis and prognosis that serves as archetype for many mutual contributions between the two. An earlier combination of these two arts classified fevers according to their periodicities. In fact principles of classification of disease have been formulated by analogy with the classification of series in mathematics. There are periodic processes, simply accelerating processes, simply decelerating processes, and significant combinations of these. Hypothetical constructions, for instance, chronaxy theory, is leading experimentation in neurology such as Adrian is now doing, as they earlier led in the study of chronic diseases.

Prognosis can be done on the larger units, the plots that need themselves to be combined into a biography. It is imaginable that something like Dr. Meyer's biographic chart might be incorporated in the hospital chart for all patients. If this were done, it would provide another standard pattern to be filled in, and a working criterion for good prognosis. Such a chart would point out the items to be sought and show the possible ways in which subplots might be subordinated to the main plot. The great advantage of this would be that there would be explicitly recognized rules for biography rather than the *ad hoc* therapeutic considerations that at present dominate and continually threaten to reduce prognosis to a mere subsidiary of therapy. Under present standards prognosis uncovers only enough of the past and future to single out one cause for all the trouble. The main objection to such reduction is that it presupposes an erroneous notion of causation, and prognosis by following this notion ends in accepting any condition that may be singled out and changed by therapy as the genuine cause. This substitution lies at the root of most modern quackery, the kind of quackery which is often accepted unawares by the honest professional man.

This is one of many points where the methods and aims of the engineering laboratory have been imitated by the medical man until he has forgotten the traditional background from which both he and the physicist have emerged. Prognosis cultivated for its own traditional ends of knowing the biography of the individual as well as of his disease, and thus maintaining a context in which the manifold data may become significant, is now left truncated at the first point which leads or seems to lead to therapeutic measures. Fully developed it might lead to deeper diagnosis and more versatile therapy.

It is true that prognosis should in the end lead to the determination of the genetic causes of disease, but there is a long route to this end and several apparent short-cuts. The weight of scientific opinion seems to be on the side of the short-cuts. Scientific societies have been known to vote for the elimination of the notion of cause from their consideration, and even when they have not gone to this extreme, they have formulated calculuses of correlation that effect the same aetiological chaos.   In the natural sciences this opinion mirrors an interesting state of affairs which will presumably in the course of time right itself.   On account of certain mathematical techniques which have become dominant as apt solutions for current technical problems the Newtonian notion of efficient cause has become obviously inadequate.   Since the scientist has been warned against formal causes by critics of medieval thought, and he has been trained in a school of science that denies all but observed things, he chooses, perhaps for good practical reasons, to drop the notion of cause altogether.   Actually he is now shifting his attention from efficient causes to formal causes which appear darkly in the mathematical formulae.   In medicine we have a less sophisticated situation.   Here efficient causes are still sought with enthusiasm and over-rated success, because the bacteriological origin of disease still holds the main aetiological position.   There are already some able heretics, even in bacteriology, but under the con- ventional demands of practice, bacteria are still the aetiological goals.   Consequently the medical man stops when he meets a bacterium, or sometimes when he anticipates meeting one.   It is said that physicians once stopped their search when they came to a sin that caused the disease, or a demon was suspected.   In principle the bacterium has taken the demon's place.   The situation may clear itself when it is realized that the bacterium also must be diagnosed and prognosed and the terminus lies through rather than in his body.

The final aetiological judgment which results from the

prognostic art will be a set of alternatives bound together in a complex dilemma under a principle, the formal cause. Efficient causes are plural and get their causal efficacy as well as their significance only from the relations they hold to one another or from the principle that governs their operation. The formal cause which performs this synthetic and interpretive function lies hidden in the biographical story. In this it is like the complex predicate of the diagnostic judgment which comes clear in the pattern of pathological alternatives. It is obvious that the ideal biography which prognosis constructs is intended to be a complicated predicate in a proposition whose subject is this sick individual. The role which prognosis studies is the role not only of a persona dramatis ; it is also the role of an individual in real life who has also taken on a character in the medical drama.

If diagnosis analyses character, and prognosis develops the plot, therapy is the action of the drama. The three arts are related as their subject-matters, and although it may seem that only the former two extend beyond the immediate scene of the action, therapy itself is best understood as also looking forward and backward when it is most intensively directed at the present. This is obviously true if we remind ourselves that therapy is applied with the aim of changing a previous course of disease to one of health, but it is more subtly true when we consider it as a contribution made by the physician to the complicated action that is taking place within the patient incessantly. Although it is artificial, it must, like all artificial processes, fit nature ; in fact, it must be natural, only more so.

There is a dangerous temptation to think of therapy as intermittent and specific, and consequently to classify measures of therapy under terms that are relevant to specific instruments, aims, and principles. Thus there might be an explorative therapy, a palliative therapy, a surgical therapy, a drug therapy, a hydrotherapy, and a mental therapy, and a description of these seriatim would seem to be a description of therapy in general. There is the same temptation in the other arts, and there is the same danger, namely that medicine shall not only be thought to be *ad hoc*, but that it shall actually become so. Therapy is one of the routes by which medicine has been specialized, and by which the specialities have become vicious. For as soon as one kind of therapy has set itself up, it tends to reduce previous practices to nonsense. Thus we get our medical cults.

The etymology of the word therapy suggests an antidote to this degenerative tendency of practical medicine. Therapy means nursing and its general working significance is given in the notion of regimen. In this light the emergency measures taken to meet acute symptoms become merely specular incidents in a course of a case, and if we are to understand them in their proper perspective we must attend to the system of therapeutic measures within which they occur. In other words we are thrown back upon the notion of a medical art as an aspect of continuous medical care, and its relation with the other arts or aspects will be indispensable in our understanding of it.

For instance it must be recalled that therapeutic measures are indicated by symptoms, and they are therefore intimately connected with diagnosis. Likewise therapeutic measures effect changes in the organism and they therefore follow upon prognosis and provide grounds for further prognosis. A great deal of therapy will not be immediately connected with the curative process itself. It may be primarily applied in order to hasten the appearance of crucial symptoms, or the production of a situation which can be judged, in other words, the crisis. Or it may aim merely to establish standard conditions both for diagnosis and further therapy. This does not imply that therapy is not ultimately directed to the end of curing, but it means that there are many-sided functions and subordinations within the curative procedures.

Perhaps the most dramatic shift in theme and manner of discussion that enters into staff conferences on cases in hospitals is the shift from the question, what is the matter with the patient, to the question what shall we do for the patient ? Each item in the diagnosis and prognosis has for the physician indicated something to be done, so that there are as many courses of action proposed as there are symptoms recorded. But here more than in any other art the implicit logic of the situation quickly condenses the chaotic possibilities to a very few practical possibilities. It is in this situation that the famous Hippocratic dictum is most dramatically significant : Life is short, the art long, judgment difficult, opportunity fleeting, the issue uncertain. These remarks are often taken to refer to the many accidental features of the medical situation which make it ambiguous and pre-carious, but their meanings easily penetrate the well analysed and controlled case where accidents are at a minimum, and they then describe at once the fine points in the actual practice of any art and the essential points in the medical art where experience, wit, and skill make necessarily swift and drastic decisions. Traditional rules have to adjust themselves to the idiosyncrasies of the special case, and this means in an analysed case that one rule must meet and adjust itself to other rules that are equally applicable. Judgment between two rules may involve some ingenious compromise or the ruthless elimination of one alternative. Each measure adopted and applied contributes its special effects to the next situation, and the omission of a measure may make an equal contribution. Ignoring the immediate crisis therefore means facing its effects in the next. What turns up as a result of a present measure determines what shall be done in the next instance. As in a tightly constructed drama there is a strict determinism demanded in a series of situations which only as they happen present alternative possibilities.

The reason for this complicated pattern can be seen in the single unit of therapy. Suppose it is the introduction of a simple measured chemical which is known to have had a specific effect. It is introduced into a system of many chemicals in the body, some known and some unknown, undergoing various changes and combinations. Besides the one known specific effect there are secondary effects some of which may be as important as the one indicated. Each of these secondary effects may set up conditions which themselves become matters for diagnosis and treatment. The chemical illustration merely typifies the many-sided significance and effects of any therapeutic measure. It was the recognition of this that led Hahnemann into the study of drugs, and from that to the perhaps exaggerated respect he developed for the unknown curative powers of nature. A thorough going system of therapy based on this point would replace physiology with a kind of mysticism or would develop a much more complicated physiology than any we have now. Homœopathy has had both effects.

We have here returned to the notion of causation and its role in the medical arts. The conscientious therapist needs no emphasis added to his knowledge of the plurality of efficient causes and the correlated plurality of effects. These seem at first to complicate the therapeutic problem, but actually in practice they present a kind of working solution. Since many of the secondary effects of therapy overlap, a knowledge of their interpenetrations reduces the number of measures required in a given circumstance and allows for a systematization of remedies in pharmacology. This is one reason that the sudden restriction of possibilities in the therapeutic phase of the medical arts comes about. It means that one measure may have a generality of effect that meets a complex pattern of symptoms and points to a single course of treatment.

One could add many other apparent complications arising from other than causal considerations. For instance, the therapeutic measure always has an experimental and explorative aspect. The effects of a drug may be equally revealing of internal states with the surgeon's knife. The mere administration of a traditional remedy may have a psychic effect and cure neurotic symptoms. All these aspects may be complications and lead to confusion or they may clarify and simplify the case. Knowledge of principle seasoned by experience makes all the difference.

What I have been saying about therapy merely parallels in other terms the things that I have said about diagnosis and prognosis, and, as the ends of these in the diagnostic judgment and in the biography were general and best expressed in alternatives, so the therapeutic end is that very complicated state called health, which is perhaps best formulated in a statement of the alternative conditions of the possibility of continued life.

CHAPTER IV

THIS running account of the three medical arts has been neither complete nor closely analytical.   I have made it because I have been unable to find any verbal statement of what happens in the hospital.   I have no doubt that it is distorted and very different from what the physician would say if he could be induced to talk or write about what for him is obvious and non-verbal.   The medical arts are for the most part like the industrial arts still passed on by practical contagion both in the later years of medical school and in the following years of internship, both of which continue the tradition of old-fashioned apprenticeship.   The philosopher, therefore, has serious difficulty in getting the kind of first level information that he needs.   Let this be an apology to the medical man for the groupings of an outsider.   I am hoping that the statement of the previous chapter, such as it is, will at least serve to illustrate the analysis that I now wish to make.

The underlying assumption in this analysis is that the clinical arts and sciences, diagnosis, prognosis, and therapeutics, take raw material, signate matter, and assimilate it to science.   The raw material is given in the case under observation and treatment, and the operations and formulations of the clinical arts and sciences bring the case under the general propositions that constitute the medical sciences. I shall have more to say about anatomy, physiology, and pathology in a later section ; it is sufficient here to recognize that these sciences contain general propositions relevant at least indirectly to the individual case.

The terms of the analysis will be the terms of the liberal arts as I have treated them in an earlier section, and in this use of them I am further assuming that the clinical arts are applications of the liberal arts to medicine just as the arts of observation, experimentation, and verification in the laboratory are applications of the liberal arts to physics. In fact, any body of scientific doctrine has a fringe of tentative exploration and operation which consists in the application of the liberal arts.

In view of the difficulty of this kind of analysis and the very complicated interpenetrations of the clinical arts, it may be well to recall briefly the main elementary distinctions that the liberal arts make. In the first place it should be clear that the liberal arts are dealing with signs and symbols, and that the distinctions they make are concerned with the diversity in their modes of signifying. Thus grammar deals with signs that point to individual concrete things, either singly or in groups ; it also deals with the artificial concrete marks and signs as they enter into combinations that constitute notations. These two modes are called respectively, first and second impositions. Grammar in its original restricted meaning deals with writing and reading, and its most characteristic concern is with translating, that combination of writing and reading which passes from one notation to another.

Grammar takes on a rhetorical aim and method as soon as two notations are well enough correlated to appear as alternative versions of what the symbols signify. Checking a translation puts the two versions in analogy with one another. Rhetoric as an art manipulates analogies and exploits their patterns of relations by expansion or condensation into figures of speech, and in so doing extends the range of the original modes of signifying. Rhetoric systematizes the correspondence between notations and consequently explores the field of their possible references, always working through analogies.

Rhetorical ordering and exploration ends in the explicit formulation of the constituent analogues, but as soon as that is accomplished the signs and symbols in the analogy have become terms in propositions. Dialectic or logic then takes over the material and explores other modes of signifying that are called first and second intentions. The terms in the propositions now refer to classes of things and are said to have first intentions ; but they also refer to abstractions or universals, and are therefore said to have second intentions. The common form in the analogy is at first merely grammatical or notational. In logical analysis a new notation is constructed that will express the common logical form abstracted from and rendered independent of any notational modes that signify particulars. Propositions so formulated express scientific principles in the light of which the original data can be understood.

I have tried to show how this analytical machinery is

used in the natural sciences as they are pursued in the laboratory. There the immediate data are usually taken to be sensations or sensa, and I chose to treat them in accordance with the rules of the liberal arts as if elements in a natural notation which could be translated into the artificial symbols of a technical language. These technical terms are then combined and systematized according to the grammatical rules of the artificial language, such translation always checked by means of instruments and new observations. This in physics ends in the making of systems of concrete numbers to express the results of the checked translation that is called measurement. These concrete numbers are then recognized as terms in analogies between mathematical formulae and observed data, and they may be expressed in the abbreviated forms that correspond to figures of speech. But formulae are more than descriptions of data. They contain principles which are discovered and reformulated as the laws of nature. Thus by translation and abstraction the crude materials of observation are assimilated to scientific abstractions as facts obeying laws.

Diagnosis, prognosis, and therapeutics are doing a similar thing to the data of medical observation. The admission of a patient to the hospital makes him a text to be read and translated into the medical languages. His symptoms are potential signs which the diagnostician has to translate into statements of the medical sciences. There will be many such symbols in a given case and they must be fitted together as words in a sentence according to the rules of what may be called a medical grammar. The difficulty in analysis begins right here, for diagnosis is an art whose science or theory is seldom made explicit. It seems that the greater the skill of the diagnostician the less explicit he is about the rules of his practice.

There are two approaches that can be suggested for this first level of medical interpretation of signs. The first is the classification of data according to the method and technique of observation. Thus gross observation and verbal report of past symptoms, laboratory tests, controlled observation with specialized instruments, exploratory medication and surgery, and bacteriological analysis present data of various kinds. Let us say that each of these modes of observation gives us a signature, such as temperature, pulse, respiration, indices for various constituents of the blood, urine, and other bodily parts, evidence of bacterial infection, etc. Each of these is ear-marked by its place of origin in the patient and the method by which it is discovered. These signatures are like words in a dictionary, and the first level classifications of the hospital chart are like the dictionary indications for the parts of speech and the possible uses the word may have.

From the side of the medical sciences there is another approach, model propositions from the subsidiary sciences into which these signatures may fit. From these two starting points the diagnostician may set out to make his translation from the concrete signs presented in the case to the descriptive medical propositions, with the aim of fitting the signatures together in sentences. Thus the pattern made up of temperature, pulse, and breathing makes what might be called a syndrome, and is destined to become an integral part of the disease picture.

Laboratory findings make up other such partial pictures.

It might seem that these pictures would fit together like the parts of a picture puzzle, but the task is not as simple as that. They belong for the most part to what in physics would be called diverse dimensions. Findings of one laboratory, such as the chemical laboratory, belong to one dimension, while findings of the bacteriological laboratory belong to another dimension, and there is no direct means for combining the two sets of findings. On the other hand, in order to be useful, these findings must be combined, and ways, if not rules, must be found for doing the combining. To a certain extent the medical sciences provide such rules since they are themselves combinations of the various sciences that dictate the observations and the laboratory tests. The combinations of physics, chemistry, and biology, that are to be found in physiology, suggest paths for the interpretation of symptoms. But these are often misleading, and a great deal depends upon the ingenuity and intuition of the diagnostician. Most of this process is no more intelligible to the lay person than the hospital chart upon which it is recorded, and both are intelligible to the physician only as he has flashes of insight to go with his execution of the professional rules.

The intuition and the ingenuity of the diagnostician are very much like the orator's sympathy with his audience and his instinct for the right word and gesture. There is a playfulness about imagination and trial-and-error thinking that seems to ignore or confuse the data. Actually the playfulness and trial-and-error thought move about within the labyrinths of the analogies that arise by the juxtaposition of syndromes. Just as figures of speech arise in discourse by the juggling of words or from day-dreaming, and afterwards reveal their roots in a complex analogy, so the syndromes derived from observation of symptoms are shuffled like cards until they reveal hidden similarities and differences that are significant for medical science. A great many analogies have to be looked into before the right one is found to serve as basis for the inductive process. Each one may have to be put through its moods and figures in order to elicit the hidden relations which appear at first only in the similarities and differences that the diagnostician feels.

It would take a great deal of painstaking study to formulate all the possible permutations and combinations that syndromes undergo in the physician's mind, but attention to the formal aspect of these would lead to something like the mathematical techniques that are used in physics. Although many syndromes are at present quantitative, they need not take that particular mathematical form in order to enter a clinical calculus. A great deal of the non-mathematical side of analogy in physics is now done by instrumental manipulation and operations that imitate imaginative trial and error, and these with the strictly mathematical calculations are but extensions and embodiments of analogical thinking. These devices of formal logic and rhetoric are never substitutes for the original endowments of genius and insight, but expansions and implementations of them. It is safe to say that medicine would not be harmed by the greater subtlety that such devices might bring. The emphasis on quantitative analysis which is now dominating medicine needs such complementary developments in the non-quantitative sphere.

The possibility of analogical interpretation in any set of data seems to evidence a vicious ambiguity in these data, and to argue for a drastic elimination of irrelevance. This is the modern reaction to processes that are recognized to be analogical, but it is not in keeping either with the actual present use of implicit analogies nor with their ancient analyses in the liberal arts. Ambiguity is vicious only because it has not been made systematic and exhaustive, and the correct theoretical rule is to save the full significance of symbols by making distinctions and rationalizing their many modes of signifying. Analogies are the proper forms within which the necessary distinction and rationalization can be made. This was so when the reading and interpretation of texts was the regular practice of scholars; it has always been the main line of development in the mathematical arts that contribute to modern scientific work. Clarification of empirical material, which is always ambiguous at first, demands good humour, patience, and enthusiasm for its meandering ways.

In diagnosis the single symptom is radically ambiguous. It belongs to many syndromes, and its only legitimate interpretation demands a thorough exploration of the possible syndromes to which it may belong. As the earlier description pointed out any given symptom is a centre from which lines of inquiry start in various directions. This can be seen in a schematic representation of syndromes in an analogical pattern. Suppose we have collected symptoms A, B, D, etc., and by rough classification they have been placed tentatively in syndromes as follows :

```
A     B         D
      F         H
I           K   L
```

In the first place we can see that the diagnosis is incomplete, and that there are more data to be obtained. The syndrome in the first row demands a third term ; the second row demands a first and third term ; and the third a second term. Observations and tests may follow this simple pattern by filling in the blanks, but more often than not the special case fails to present the expected data. It may then be noted that the analogical pattern of the scheme above shows other possible syndromes and combinations of symptoms which determine vertical lines of inquiry complementary to the former horizontal lines. Thus we may say that one column demands a second term and its connection with A and I may be more suggestive of the sort of finding wanted than the second row had been. It goes without saying that this use of the analogical pattern is merely for the purpose of discovery and should not be laid on dogmatically in such a way as to prevent a complete re-arrangement if unexpected data are found. It is useful even in such a circumstance since it allows a clear judgment of fitness or unfitness.

However, there is another use of the same scheme when the aim is to integrate the picture as a whole. By the alternate tracing of rows and columns with the aim of finding definite and unambiguous relations between the symptoms, the implicitness of the analogy gives way to explicit statement of symptoms in defined relationships, which are called nosograms. This transformation of syndromes into nosograms represents another step towards the physiological and pathological propositions that are sought. Nosograms are syndromes that show their inner connections, and it is in this final formulation that the analogical scheme delivers its rows and columns in tight relational patterns. The previous analogical ambiguities condense, crystallize, and break up into analytical statements that are amenable to abstract physiological interpretation.

The clarification thus brought about has been due to many bits of analysis, ranging from the sort that is characteristic of common sense to highly technical theoretical analysis in the sciences. The range can be seen in the interpretations of the X-ray photograph. It may be that a gross finding of palpation is to be compared with the X-ray picture of a given region ; the common-sense knowledge of geometry will suffice to correlate the data of touch with the shadows on the plate. On the other hand, it may be that the X-ray photograph is to verify the microscopic findings of the histologist and his microscope ; in this case a knowledge of sub-atomic physics will be necessary to bridge the dimensions involved. Such comparisons and correlations fill in the gaps in the analogical schema and the tight pattern of terms is a nosogram, which now looks like this transformation of the original syndromal pattern :

A	r	B	r	C	r	D
r		r		r		r
E	r	F	r	G	r	H
r		r		r		r
I	r	J	r	K	r	L

The original schema, of course, may have been revised and re-arranged in more complex relations with more terms added.

At this point the Sydenham school of empirical diagnosis would make a diagnostic judgment in a proposition of which the patient is the subject and the nosogram is the complex predicate. The nosogram would be the disease and the judgment would say that this patient has it. Pathology would in this context be the science which classifies nosograms and the body of knowledge to which it would point would be a museum of nosography. Physiology would presumably be a similar museum of normograms.

But for a more rationalistic school of diagnosis nosograms have to be still further transformed. The analogical patterns have to be broken up and reformulated in propositions that would compendently belong to a medical science. The general propositions in these sciences have already been turned into hypothetical models and guides for the construction of nosograms and syndromes. The syndromes have been variations on these basic patterns, or, if you like, the given symptoms have been trial values substituted for the variables in these general propositions. It is in these hypothetical models that the rows and columns of the nosograms appear as empirical propositions describing concrete data. Given symptoms in a syndrome have been shuffled and fitted to the abstract content of various general propositions, and their correlation has gone on in the resulting analogies. The discovery or clarification of the nosograms consists in the definite determination of the relative positions of symptoms in the syndromes in the scheme, and vice versa the arrangement of them in the scheme has helped in the discovery of their explicit relations. The final step is the separation of rows and columns and their formulation in abstract physiological and pathological propositions which in their first intention will still be descriptive of the case.

On one side this demands reference of the constituent terms in the nosograms to the classes within which they fall, according to strictly medical categories. Propositions are expressed as sentences in which there are subjects, predicates, and copulas, and the copulas, forms of the verb "to be", connect subjects and predicates in various categorical ways, which have been matter for logical analysis throughout the history of philosophy. The medical categories are special cases of more general categories and at various times have had more explicit attention than they have at present in medical and philosophical thought. I shall treat this subject more at length in a later section in connection with more strictly physiological problems. It will be sufficient here to outline the approach to the needed methods of classification.

We have our material in the large variety of relations that hold signatures together in nosograms. Our aim is to arrive at strictly physiological and pathological propositions which have determinate positions in these sciences, so that at least for pragmatic purposes the whole of the medical sciences can be brought to bear on the case under observation and treatment. We need some intermediary terms and arrangements to effect this transformation.   At present such terms and arrangements are given in the physiological accounts of the skeletal, circulatory, nervous, gastro-intestinal, and endocrine systems.   It is in these systematic accounts that the nosographic relations should fit, and whatever the highest generalities are in these accounts they are the medical categories.   These systems serve the same purpose for present physiology that Galenic faculties served in Galenic medicine.

The propositions that result from this assimilation will be special determinations or specifications of the most general propositions that determine these abstract systems.   The nosograms are still values substituted in these general equations, but they have now lost their status as trial values.   The systems are applied and the values are fixed.   The set of such propositions is the complex predicate of the diagnostic judgment which the physician has been working to make.   Therefore the set is expressed in a group of interdependent propositions linked together in hypothetical, disjunctive, and con- junctive propositions.   This set taken as a system becomes the predicate of a single elementary proposition such as " John, the patient before us, has typhoid fever ".   This is the diagnostic proposition which the physician asserts, its predicate containing systematically all the complexi- ties of the analysis he has made.

This last step from nosograms to propositions in medical science marks the passage from rhetoric to logic in diagnosis.

Even in a quick diagnosis where the final judgment leaps to the eye, in addition to the materials presented for observation there are also preconceptions in the mind of the diagnostician which play an essential part in the process of judgment.   It was earlier remarked that these preconceptions are ordered in a genus-species hierarchy, and that the mind of the physician moves about among these according to the rules of logic.   The actual movements are made through the analogical forms of rhetorical thought, but these in their turn are imitating the logical prototypes which could be handled with syllogisms and the traditional devices of formal logic.   The passage from syndromes through nosograms to propositions marks an actual movement from analogies to traditional forms of subsumption and inference.   Although the applied aspect of physiology is uppermost in the mind of the physician in his treatment of the case, still the abstractions are the immediate subject-matter of the medical propositions derived from the nosograms, and the aim even at this stage is to render the propositions consistent within themselves and externally with each other.   To a great extent the tests for consistency will be by rule of thumb, that is by seeing if the propositions derived from the nosograms conform with their models in the science itself, but there will often be propositions that have no precedents in physiology.   In such cases there will be a dilemma, either to revise physiology or to correct the new propositions.   It is under the discipline of such dilemmas that physiology grows from the clinical source, and it is on account of them that problems are passed on to the laboratory.   The practising physician has his choice and for the most part will revise and correct his observations to fit established physiology as far as possible, but there will often be impressive reasons for revising his physiology on the spot.   In so doing he is contributing to medical science, just as the judge in the court is making law when he faces a conflict of laws and makes a new decision.

The trivial analysis of the propositions of a science such as physiology to show the distinctions between their first and second intentions, their descriptive and abstract references, nicely contributes to the double aim of the diagnostician.   He must find out what is the trouble with the patient before him, and he must also make available for the patient the intelligibility that lies in the abstractions of the medical sciences.   The details of the patient's troubles have been isolated and explored according to the grammatical and rhetorical rules of diagnosis.   The logic of diagnosis comes through the propositions of physiology when they are understood as the formulation of abstractions and their connections.   This understanding consists in grasping the second intention of the terms and seeing the necessities of their connections.   But the same terms also represent classes of things, and their logical connections and oppositions in abstracto correspond to the inclusions and exclusions of these classes.   Second intentions exhibit the reasons hidden in the association of concrete things, and through them the complex pattern of symptoms gains an intelligible unity or explanation. Classes in such orderly unities are the first intentions of the scientific propositions.   With first and second intentions thus established the detailed troubles of the patient can be distinguished, arranged, and subsumed in the classes and their complicated relations become intelligible in the principles of physiology. It is thus that the scattered rays that arise from the analysis of the individual patient are collected and focused in a physiological insight.

It is impossible in the serial form of exposition, that I am attempting, to point out all the points or regions of overlapping and interpenetration of the clinical arts. The respective domains of diagnosis and prognosis are related much as space and time are related in physics. There is activity and change at any point and the diagnostic analysis stops the process and fixes its elements with the distortion usually incident to static illusions. On the other hand, it is impossible to talk sense in science without this distortion ; in fact style in science consists in the static transfiguration. As I have said before, excellence in science is to be achieved only by realizing the special virtues or potentialities in it. Consequently, if diagnosis is static in its results, its potentialities in this direction should be cultivated and realized. Similarly in prognosis the characteristic temporal feature should be exhaustively explored and utilized, but since prognosis contributes to medical science, it will itself turn out results that are static in the end. In fact, there are two main themes to be developed in an analysis of prognosis, one based on the temporal patterns discovered in the case and even these will turn into static diagnostic patterns ; and the other the dynamic set of natural operations which are closely comparable with the operations of therapeutics.

The elementary task of prognosis is therefore the transformation of a continuous change into a series of stages. The first step in this transformation is the building of a chronology of the case in which each event will be an item related to those that come before and those that come after it in a temporal series. Here, as in the case of diagnosis, the elementary units that go into the series will be symptoms which have the usual properties of signatures, namely the capacity of fitting into syndromes, or grammatical patterns. In some case these patterns will already have been supplied by diagnosis, but the distinguishing mark of a prognostic nosogram will be the introduction of temporal relations to bind the symptoms together. The grammar of prognosis will be found in the application of time schemes. These may be recorded in numbers representing rhythmical rates as in pulse and respiration, or they may be of higher scale as in the temperature, pulse, and respiration charts that show the rhythmical rise and fall of these rates over a period of hours or days. Or they may be of still higher scale as in recurrent fevers or chronic diseases marked by acute attacks at longer measured intervals. These are characteristic simple cases of prognostic syndromes.

As the observed symptoms supply prognostic signatures for the elementary syndromes, so these syndromes in their turn supply the material that is combined in syndromes of the next higher order of complexity. Time still supplies the order according to which the constituent syndromes are combined, and the resulting combinations begin to look like histories, or episodes in the history of the disease process. It is on this level that the prognostician begins to look for the entity that is undergoing the change, the disease entity, the bacterium, the organ system, etc. Any literal-minded search for such an entity is hardly justified, but the tendency to make such a search is understandable, since the process shows a constancy of form with a change in material. In fact, the disease process seen in this pattern seems to mimic metabolism. The form of one syndrome becomes the archetype for the others, and as they are ordered in time, it appears that the symptoms come and go displacing and replacing one another in the pattern as chemical units do in the metabolism of the cell. Many irrelevant suggestions follow. Some of these can be symbolized in Lewis Carroll's parody of Mill's methods. For instance, consider the clinical account of the passage of meat into stew in the following pattern :

M E A T
S E A T
S E A M
S E E M
S T E M
S T E W

Each word makes a syndrome. Repetition of letters suggests persistence of symptoms and clues to causes ; E looks like a preponderant cause ; E may be the effect of a bacterium. M looks like a genetic cause whose elimination or prevention would result in health. But just as the alphabet, phonetics, and the acrostic are not the clue to the proper playing or understanding of the game, so Mill's methods and statistics miss the point. The game works only for him who sees the identity of form, in this case, four letter word, and divines the rule of

one-letter substitution.   In the light of these observation
and operation become significant, and not otherwise.

It was some such pattern that struck the early
diagnosticians and led up to the so-called Hippocratic
study of disease processes with the hope that a single
prognostic form could be discovered for all diseases.
This point has been over-emphasized by students of the
Hippocratic writings, but it has nonetheless been a
constant theme in medicine since that time.   Initial
disturbance, complication, coction, crisis, and abscession
are never wholly absent from the context of the prognostic
art, and they serve to mark the stages in disease histories
even when they are not mentioned.   The bacteriological
theory of disease, with its stages of infection, incubation,
onset, crisis, formation of antibodies, and final immuniza-
tion gives the current generalization of the historical
prognostic model.   These are merely ordinal names for
the successive syndromes in the prognostic series.

It should be pointed out for the purposes of our analysis
that the syndromes are analogues of one another, and
that, like the analogues in the diagnostic picture, there
are lines of correspondence between the respective terms.
But in addition to the lines of correspondence we have
here the line of temporal order connecting analogue with
analogue, and therefore term with term.   In fact the
prognostic picture is a rearrangement of the diagnostic
syndromes to allow the introduction of the temporal
relations between them.   This does not mean that the
re-arrangement is of slight importance, for it is one of the
efficient ways of insuring that the syndromal analogies
are well shuffled and explored.   Time relations suggest

and lead to the discovery of all sorts of genetic relations and finally push the prognostician to the ordering of causes under the principles of physiology, which even as an abstract science is concerned with processes of time.

But the prognosis of disease is not safe or complete until the disease history has been placed in the patient's biography.   The construction of such a biography follows the lines laid down by the disease history, but in extending the range of relevant data, it serves to check the immediate data, and to revise notions of normal process to fit the individual and his idiosyncrasy.

The final biographical picturé is like the inside of a cylindrical tunnel through which the individual has lived, leaving the record of his living on its internal walls, and the prognostic chart in its ideal form would be the inside of the cylinder unrolled and spread out for the diagnostician to read.

The logic of prognosis is identical with that of diagnosis. Implicit relations in syndromes are rendered explicit in nosograms and formulated in terms of physiological laws, which themselves become complex systematic predicates of the subject of the diagnostic judgment, namely the patient.   The entities of disease and the causes of disease are finally physiological entities and causes.

It is only at the end of our analysis of prognosis that we have a right to talk about it in its original sense as foreknowledge within which predictions can be based. In the history of medicine this order would be reversed. The pre-professional doctor or physician had to persuade his patients that he had the knowledge and skill to deal with their troubles, and he used his medical knowledge in its most spectacular form as it bore on the future to demonstrate his ability.   Prediction is the most impressive of rhetorical devices when the audience is composed of self-styled practical men.   It has high persuasive value, and in social matters it has the apparently magical power of helping to verify itself.   There are on record cases of men who died because they were told they were going to die, as well as the suggestive cases of men who recovered because they were told they were not sick.   Prediction is thus a part of therapy, and to discuss it as part of prognosis is to introduce the part of prognosis that is most clearly connected with therapy.

There are a great many more sciences and a great many more parts of sciences than are usually recognized that proceed by construction rather than observation in their empirical investigations.   This constructive aspect of science is often discussed under the heading " fictions in science ", and has a large literature since the time of Jeremy Bentham, who invented a corresponding method for the criticism of modern science.   The tone of most of this literature is negatively critical, as may be seen in the phrase " necessary fiction ", which is obviously modelled on the phrase " necessary evil ".   However, all this literature admits the necessity of fictions in science, and to a certain degree it demonstrates the functions that fictions can perform.   The Baconian apology for science is the only clear case of a serious claim that science can do without fictions, and I think we can credit the claim to the Lord Chancellor's penchant for rhetorical ruses.

The science of mathematics very early in its modern renaissance not only admitted its fictional character, but

claimed a plenipotentiary license in the matter of constructions. From the empirical point of view points and
straight lines are clearly fictions, and so are numbers and
algebraic variables, and these are only the building blocks
of a vast speculative edifice. The philosopher who is
aware of his traditional background sees in this a
backswing of the pendulum which moves between the
limiting extremes of rationalism and empiricism. It is
only in a predominantly empirical period of thought
that the expressions for ideas and principles are called
fictions and are accused of being made up out of whole
cloth.

Thus it becomes the duty of the philosopher to point
out that predictions in any science are fictions, and further
to point out that scientific authorities who are wary of
both predictions and fictions are unaware of the second
intention of the terms that they are using. Whether they
like it or not, their terms and their descriptive factual
propositions have second intentions, refer to universal
terms that go beyond the facts, and even have bearing
on the non-existent future. Thus a thorough prognostic
analysis of the data in a case not only establishes a history
of that case, but at the same time it predicts a future
with a certain degree of probability. But more important
than the mere prediction is the regulative effect of the
abstractions that have been educed from the material.
The prediction leads to the search for new data by laying
down the alternative possibilities for the future of the
case. As soon as the possibility of prediction arises in
the analysis of a case there is evidence that we are dealing
however blindly and fumblingly with universals that

belong to science, and if we have doubts about fictions we may as well give in to them at least as far as to say that it is on their wings that we have risen to the consideration of scientific truths.

Nevertheless, it may be well to look into the origin of these fictional processes and see if that will give the empiricist some reassurance that he is not being fooled when he becomes a scientist unawares. The origin of fictions is in the constructions that go into the artificial making of science, and the mathematicians have led the way by an analysis of such constructions into their elements, which they call operations. Thus in diagnosis I have tried to show that the first steps are translations of the concrete symptoms presented by the patient into the terms of technical language which is *par excellence* an artificial linguistic construction. Even here we have the operation of substituting an artificial sign for a natural product, and as soon as this is done by giving a thing a name, we immediately proceed to combine it with other names according to the rules of a grammar. Out of the elementary linguistic units we build higher units, the syndromes. These in turn are still further combined according to rule of thumb or rule of grammar, and the constructive process goes on until we have the full explicit nosogram. Similarly in prognosis we have the construction of an artificial or ideal biography according to the rules of the prognostic art. It is by something very closely akin to calculation in mathematics that we arrive at the scientific propositions that we wish to bring to bear on the case. The mathematician speaks of a set of operations as a transformation, and I have been using his language when I have spoken of the transformation of signatures into science.

We have something here that reminds us of the incantations of primitive medicine. These were the rules for the connecting of signatures with remedies, as modern science does in a more analytic and explicit way. Science as a set of abstractions and corresponding operations is said to keep closer to the facts, and the meaning of this is that the scientist by his actual physical operations keeps his abstractions in closer step with the operations that nature performs for him. Thus in medicine science improves therapy, and in turn therapeutic operations contribute to science. In a very profound sense the intellect knows only what the hand does.

I do not think it is necessary further to labour the point that operations are being performed in every step of the diagnosis and prognosis of a case, and that the operations with symbols, which lead towards the understanding, are always in correspondence with the operations that lead to the more obvious therapeutic end of curing disease. The analogy here is of the essence of good therapy and good empirical science. It will be better to turn to a more subtle and perhaps a more profound point. If we take natural and therapeutic operations together and consider them in the same context with experimental techniques, we may recognize in them the origin of the most important modern mode of achieving intellectual insights in science. The experiment has historically risen from medical therapy, and both belong, as far as their philosophical consideration is concerned, to the part of philosophical doctrine that treats of practical reason. It is therefore somewhat of an anomaly that scientists pride themselves on their pure interest in fact and law and their independence of practical concerns. The French words for experiment and experience, whose English equivalents have been so widely exploited in the defence of British-American empiricism and pragmatism, have kept most of their original connotation. They refer to the rules by which empirical data are transformed and rendered rational by technical operations, and it is assumed that anything humanely useful must be at least implicitly rational. The arts, useful, liberal, and fine, being human activities directed to ends, are therefore the expression of reason by means of human operations. Likewise the use of scientific instruments and laboratory equipment is reason at work, scientific instruments are embodiments of ideas, and their manipulation in observation and measurement is an art practised according to rational rules. Facts on one hand and laws of nature on the other are products of reason at work, and the end as well as the guide in research is understanding. There is something peculiarly European about these statements ; they appear dogmatic and stuffily traditional to the American scientific man who likes to think of himself as an intellectual pioneer stumbling on facts as he goes " with gun and camera through the alimentary canal ". If he looked closely at the guns and cameras of the laboratory, he would realize that they betray him to the rationalists of the European tradition, and that if he wishes to add science to his technology, it may be wise to capitulate and recognize the funded rationality in his tools.

The readings on a thermometer and the graduations on a flask are notational elements and the operations of taking a temperature or measuring a fluid transfer these signs to the material. These measured states and materials then become signs of still other things by similar operations. In other words instruments have first and second impositions by which the rational rules in the mind of the operator are projected into the unknown material, and as this projection progresses from one thing to another, scientific entities are created. This creation is not wholly a nominalistic affair, since practical uses of many things regularly make those things what they are. A chair and a table are what they are because we use them that way. Similarly a rigid bar becomes a lever when we move it on a fulcrum, and a poison becomes a remedy when we administer it according to a rule. Further, it is not only articles destined for human utility that are made by operations ; dirt and waste and disease are also created by operations that exclude them from use or existence. On first thought there may be some doubt about the power of words in creating things, but the creativeness of operations should be a commonplace in a world which is so thoroughly created by the industrial arts as ours is. But, magic aside, all that is necessary for us to recognize is that operations give names to things and then build them into symbolic structures. It is in this way that fictions come into science.

As soon as the operations become systematic and ordered in groups according to their effective harmonies, they can be transferred from human hands to non-human bodies, which then become tools and machines which may be able to imitate talking and calculation if they are graduated and calibrated according to human custom. They then are scientific instruments and give back rules for operations that can be performed through them for the naming and measuring of still other things. We have in this process a kind of non-human rhetoric which is surprisingly effective in its persuasiveness. Scientific instruments are machines that have so well " learned " their lessons that they can " persuade " nature to deliver up its secrets which then persuade men. It is no wonder that American scientists have developed enthusiasm for collecting facts and learning laws with this impressive set of automatons put at their beck and call, and that they speak of the subjection of nature by human art. Neither is it any wonder that the machines have gone beyond the intellects that have created them, so that now we are not sure we understand what the oracles of the laboratory are saying.

All of this is an old story to the medical profession. Therapeutic operations probably started with the aim to cure, but before the cure was effected, the operations had performed their informative function for the physician. The preconception in the mind of the physician had been refuted, verified, or modified by ordeal of operative trial. Then there were intentional trial operations apparently resulting in a flood of illuminating insights. Periodically the operations outran the rules, and therapy degenerated to magic and quackery. There is a cycle of therapeutics that rises and grows from the introduction of any new therapeutic device, and it corresponds to the kind of imaginative exploration that goes on in diagnosis. A new tool and its operations become the clue to the whole of medicine and it takes time and patience to allow it to find its context and specific powers.

Here, as usual, the road to clarity lies through the confusion rather than around it. A new therapeutic device, a new instrument, a new machine, or a new idea has to be put in motion in a material before it reveals its limitations and its range of significance and power, and the resulting confusions are places to look for the boundaries. C. S. Peirce once wrote an article for the *Scientific Monthly* entitled "How to Make our Ideas Clear". His advice was, given an idea, to look for the corresponding rule which would direct action toward the discovery of the concrete things that the idea designated. This gospel has since become the truth vouchsafed to the pragmatists, and the article is often quoted by them. It remains for the post-pragmatic critic to point out the remaining part of the scholastic doctrine from which Peirce took his text. This point should be made in an article written for some current scientific magazine entitled, "How to Find out What Facts Mean". Its advice would be to look for the rule according to which a human being might have created the actual pattern of facts and which will at the same time direct thought toward the discovery of an idea that the facts exemplify. The scholastic doctrine from which both of these advices come is that every nature whether an idea in the human mind or principle in things has its appropriate operation, and that the statement of the rule for this operation is the means by which we pass back and forth between ideas and things.

The confusion which results from the use of the non-human rhetorical devices, such as instruments and machines, according to the advice of C. S. Peirce, can only be clarified by following the complementary advice, namely to look for the rules of the operations performed with these instruments and machines, and to formulate them so that they express the abstraction that led to their use. These in the case of therapeutic operations will be the abstractions of physiology and the other adjunct medical sciences, and the therapeutic operations which seemed to be artificial will prove, in so far as they are effective and rational, to be of like nature with the natural physiological changes in the organism. Anything that the operations effect besides this will prove to be irrelevant. But these things cannot be known without the criteria provided by abstract physiological theory, which will need a special study and reformulation in a special notation which make deduction, calculation, and verification possible.

There is a very interesting case of this sort of confusion and need of clarification at present. The problem was proposed by Claude Bernard in his discussion of *le milieu intérieur*, and the attention due to it has been postponed for almost two generations because of the interest in the rival problems of bacteriology. Claude Bernard found that the balances between the various constituents of the blood were very much like the balances of potentials in an isolated electric field or in the pressures, temperatures, and volumes of gases. The facts regarding the blood were ascertained and combined by the usual means, observations, measurements, and the traditional techniques of controlled experiments. Then rhetoric of instruments had " persuaded " the blood, and it had revealed the invariant properties of its nature.

Claude Bernard took the next step, which was to assume the blood as a set of constant conditions environing the parts of the body, and he saw in this constancy the sort of controls that are demanded in laboratories built by man. In other words the environment afforded by the blood constituted the ideal constant conditions for experimentation. This was for him, with his French training in the tradition of practical reason, the solution of the difficulties that biologists pointed out as excuses for their failures in research. Nature in the living organism had provided the conditions which in other sciences had to be supplied from outside. He generalized the principle as the constancy of the internal environment, and proposed that it is at the same time one of those principles of physiology that give it a rational status.

As I suggested, it is only recently that the principle has had proper attention paid to it. The occasion for its revival has been the new problems of endocrinology and neurology. So far the interest in the principle has taken the form of search for other cases of the constancy in other physiological systems, and also of a more thorough study of the blood itself. Such searches have been combined in the work of the biochemist.

In spite of very remarkable discoveries this subject is in a peculiar state of confusion, shown in part by the riot of specialization it indulges in, and in part by the crude generalization that it suffers in the hands of the popularizer of medical knowledge, and the equally popular vogue of new cults of therapy. The confusion has at present achieved a name, homœostasis. An historical and a philosophical word of caution may be in season.

In the first place homœostasis is the name for something that is very familiar in all natural science, the constancy of form in a changing material. A great many homœostases were discovered and analysed and formulated before the name was known. Morphological anatomy is one of the sciences into which the physiologist puts them when he feels fairly sure that they will maintain themselves. The science of physiology whenever it does a good job of analysis and formulation contributes homœostases to this collection. The new specimens have drawn particular attention because they have resulted from the application of new instruments and techniques borrowed from physics and chemistry. Many of these techniques go beyond the intellects that have launched them and operate them, and homœostasis is a good general term for patterns of signatures that are not yet understood specifically.

This is the philosopher's diagnosis, and the prognosis is that physiology will go on discovering cases of such constancies, and as they accumulate, each will be better understood through the accompanying processes of analogical reasoning and the abstraction of the common properties. The philosopher's therapeutic advice is to analyse and formulate the rules for the operations that deal with homœostatic phenomena with the aim of finding the abstract principles that act in all such processes, and for the more efficient execution of this task Galenic medicine is prescribed, a matter that I shall discuss in the following section.

The logical or trivial analysis of the therapeutic arts may be concluded in a few statements about rules and abstract propositions. Rules are usually stated in imperative sentences and seem to have an exclusively particular or individual incidence on a given situation. This is so when they are rhetorically used to bring about the execution of a command, but they are, strictly speaking, not rules unless they have a general reference. Genuine rules have many cases, and therefore go beyond the immediate occasion. In cases of such and such a kind do so and so ; this is the form they take. This can further be shown by the classification into which rules fall. They may be directions for a narrow class of cases, in which case, following Kant, they are rules of skill and are often unstated because they are carried out by habit rather than by thought. Others may be hypothetical, if such and such is the case, or if such and such has been done, then do so and so. Still others may be disjunctive or alternative : in such and such a case, do either this or that. Finally, they may be categorical which amounts to the rule that applies to all cases ; in therapy such a rule might read : In all cases fit the rule or operation to the conditions, or treat each case as an individual.

The book of rules for medical therapy would make an interesting material for the philosophical analysis of medical thought, and it would probably lead to very interesting and perhaps important physiological generalizations. These rules would be general propositions, sometimes of a very high order of abstraction, and their translation into abstract propositions of physiology would undoubtedly contribute to the rationalization of our physiological knowledge. Unfortunately, therapy is the least articulate verbally of the medical arts. It is time for the thorough-going operationalist to turn his attention to it. We now have such operationalists in mathematics, physics, chemistry, astronomy and geology, and they have said significant, if at first puzzling, things about the relations between data, laws, and methods. Therapy is a most apt subject-matter for the next attempt.

CHAPTER V

THE passage from the clinical arts and sciences to the strictly medical sciences may well be eased by a few words concerning the relations between them.   In the first place, I have tried to show that the exercise of the clinical arts on the raw material proper to them has as its end the transformation of confused and ambiguous data into the clearly formulated propositions of a rational science. This means that at the start we have the tangled flux of nature or experience, and at the end we have general propositions claiming consideration as laws of nature. The clinical arts and sciences in a great variety of subtle ways carry the professional mind across the problematic territory that lies between these two extremes.   The analysis that I have tried to demonstrate seems to show that the clinical arts are special cases of the more general and perhaps universal arts that were once called liberal. Grammarian and scholar, laboratory worker and theoretician, the medical clinician and researcher are thus always partaking of and contributing to the great tradition of European thought.   The emphasis that I have made would seem to show that these arts are the ordered and tried ways by which intellectual light is always brought to focus on novel, chaotic, and puzzling concrete material.   Perhaps it would be more in keeping with the modern temper if it were admitted that the greatest efficiencies in these arts, though perhaps not the highest excellences of these arts, are at present achieved in journalism, where the run of events is caught and given a modicum of intelligibility by the rapid writing of the regular reporter on a newspaper. The translation of event into printer's ink is the most imposing practice of the liberal arts that we know about, and it is perhaps most imposing because the present moving world of action and accident actually gets into written language in this case. In the case of the grammarian and scholar there is a laboured process of translation from one language to another, and conscience and fidelity to tradition slows and narrows the work. In the laboratory where the canons of measurement seem to take the place of literary and moral controls the translation produces an esoteric text subject to continuous refinement and extension. The physician has to fulfil all these criteria of excellence, speed, conscientiousness, and modern scientific refinement. In each case, even for the journalist and the physician, it is true that life is short and the art long, and it is only the truth that will render the art liberal.

But truth demands more than skill and liberality. Somewhere and some time, however distant from the actual working artist, there is an abstract and traditional body of doctrine which acts as reservoir and also as criterion for what the scholar artist produces. His contribution and his practice must ultimately and continually be judged, and the judgment is not finally made in terms of morals, speed, refinement, nor in terms of any other criterion than abstract truth. In other stages of our tradition this ultimate criterion has been recognized and fulfilled in explicit pronouncements of dogma through established authorities. In contemporary terms it is met and fulfilled in the voluntarily accepted dogma of democratic philosophy that theory and practice shall be concerned with real things. As is usual in other applications of democratic dogma there is considerable doubt and debate concerning the status of the real things and the natures imputed to them ; nevertheless, there is a kind of working verbal agreement that whatever the selection and imputation may be the results will be called facts. Facts will be respected and fictions and artificiality will be eliminated.

There is in this agreement a good workmanlike respect for workmanship, since facts are things done either by workman or by nature, and there is also an assurance that facts will be relevant factors in the arts. As a matter of fact this is no assurance that real things will be wrung dry of all fiction and artificiality, but rather a resolution that still other criteria of truth will be respected. Factuality is a workman's as well as the scientist's shorthand word for all the metaphysical considerations that contribute to the validation of scientific truth. I shall not plunge into an exposition of the systematic details such as consistency, substantiality, generality, etc., although there is at present a great need for such an exposition for modern science in general. I shall choose another route which I hope will be more seductive and suggestive for the present state of affairs in the sciences.

This route begins to appear in a reversal of the picture that I have made of the liberal or clinical arts contributing to the store of scientific knowledge. This store of abstract wisdom is a reservoir from which the practising physician or artist draws the rules for his practice. This is obviously true in the case of therapy, but it is even more importantly true in the case of diagnosis and prognosis. I have emphasized the theoretical or speculative ends for which these arts are practised, but they also have their practical ends. The physician wishes to understand the case, the physicist wishes to abstract the laws of his phenomena, the grammarian and logician wish to interpret the text, but all of these also wish to re-apply the knowledge which they thus gain. The physician aims to cure the disease, the physicist, however modestly, wants to aid the engineer, and the scholar wishes to educate or persuade his fellows. The liberal and clinical arts might have a very different looking exposition if the expositor started with this point of view and attitude. The data in hand would then be abstractions and forms which were to be introduced into a material, and the chief concern would be to find the intermediate means for this process. The result would be a change wrought in nature and a good achieved. The artist would then be a curer of disease, a director of industry, or a statesman. In this case the genuineness of the art and science that have gone into the acts would be tested by the goodness of the results and the efficiencies of the practice. These criteria are by no means irrelevant to the science, although it is often forgotten that the application of them is as subtle and difficult as the application of the criteria of truth and reality.

The demands for efficiency and goodness thus placed on medicine must be met, if they are met at all adequately, by the medical sciences. In short these sciences must be true and useful. There is, nevertheless, considerable doubt both in the profession and from the public whether the present formulations and understandings of these sciences do fulfil these demands. The doubts are not wholesale and condemnatory, but they are nonetheless serious and sometimes intelligently specific. They are voiced whenever it appears that some relevant data are not interpreted and used, or when new development in the sciences is not smoothly and intelligently absorbed. Both of these classes of failure are well represented in day-to-day practice and research in medicine.

There are even more serious criticisms from a more detached and non-professional source. It seems that the physics which the medical man adheres to in his basic habits is the physics of two hundred years ago, so that present medical applications of contemporary physics amount to a wholesale reduction of up-to-date knowledge to out-of-date modes of thought. The anachronism in itself is not fatal, but the misunderstandings arising from misplaced context and mistaken applications are not only immediate miscarriages of knowledge, they are productive of pseudo-science and quackery, and permanent dangers to intellectual navigation. But anachronisms are only special cases of a wider array of dangers. Without a basis of comprehensive understanding of science, the medical man becomes merely a mimicker of the sciences that he tries to use. So some of the best modern medicine appears on examination to be a polyglot accumulation of superficial transcripts from other sciences, and the profession as a whole at present shows a hunger for novelty in ideas and gadgets which usually evidences the decay of the bases upon which discrimination depends.

A list of the metaphors which when taken literally have provided the basis for research, theorizing, and therapy would make up a gallery of scientific and philosophical horrors.

> The body is a system of levers.
> The body is a heat engine.
> The body is a chemical factory.
> The body is a dynamo.
> The body is a storage battery.
> The body is a radio receiving and broadcasting set.
> The body is a plant that runs on sun power.
> The body is a colony of cells.
> The body is a textile of tissues.
> The body is a writing, reading, and calculating machine.
> The body is a clock.

As I write these down, I experience the confusion and the loss of direction that conditions all the physiological thought of the present period. Each of these represents a brilliant insight and a programme of research, in some cases the establishment of a new science, but there is no end to the array and no system by which they are to be made mutually intelligible. I could shorten the list by reduction of one to a special case of another, or I could reduce the other to the one. I could accept one as fundamental and the others would then become derivative. Or I could accept one or two and condemn the rest as fictions and moonshine. I see no reason for doing one of these manipulations rather than another, except possibly personal aesthetic tastes or the conviction that I know less of some than I do of the others. I could do a trivial analysis of the metaphors and show their analogical connections and abstract the thread of reasoning that might bind them together. I might then have a consistent though somewhat fantastic dogmatic system of medicine, but it would not appeal to any one of the scientists represented here as even amusing ; it would be poison to the constructive scientific work that is going on. It is difficult to see how the discussions and controversies that arise from this tower of Babel would even please the liberal who wishes a meeting of minds, free exploration, and tolerance of heresy. The only sane thing for a scientist to do under these circumstances is unfortunately to pursue some single highly specialized point in one of the programmes here presented. That is the only sense in which we can say that the present medical laboratory worker is sane and his art valuable.

Contemplating this situation the philosopher is tempted to bold measures, and in a certain sense he is justified, or one might say compelled, to yield to the temptation. There is little hope of the good scientist, who is minding his own specialized business, devoting himself to the broken foundations of his science ; it would be only bad betting for him as an individual to give up his time and energy to a critical and general speculative investigation, when he has before him the possibility of pushing his specialty a few solid steps ahead. Then, too, the philosopher knows that the trouble with physiology is to a greater extent than is generally recognized due to historical crises in his own field which have never been properly met by his philosophical brethren. Professor Whitehead is the only modern philosopher who has recently faced this problem and dared to enter the speculative field as both scientist and philosopher. His solidly conceived criticism of physiology and his diagnosis in terms of the philosophical conceptions that lie back of it must be well known. His own reconstruction of the philosophy of science to meet the situation is probably not as well known, partly because it has in it elements of novelty that demand the invention of a new and difficult terminology, and partly because what is glimpsed through this terminology by the ordinary reader looks like an uncritical return to the speculative vagaries of the past whose elimination at the beginning of the modern period resulted in a violent scientific antipathy to anything that resembled them. This was a catastrophe whose fatality for traditional thought is only now beginning to be realized. I see no choice now for the philosopher, who must be even on the lowest standard of professional competence an historian of ideas, but to begin the slow laborious task of recalling and rebuilding the system of ideas that once made physiology a genuine science and a trustworthy basis for medical research and practice. This does not mean that I am offering the medical profession a choice between ancient and modern medicine, but rather that I am reminding it of the background and the foundation which made modern advances possible. Affairs in physiology have been running on their own momentum and on borrowings from other sciences for two hundred years at least : its rational foundation has been showing signs of decay for about a hundred years ; and a day of accounting is fast approaching. It goes without saying that all the natural sciences have been suffering from a similar decay and consequent inflations and deflations which in their influence on medicine have accelerated the degenerative processes in physiology itself.

Daremberg, the French translator of some of the most important works of Galen, makes this comment on the effect of the Renaissance in the scientific tradition : " This substitution (examination for authority), excellent in itself, but often unintelligent and too precipitous, has condemned the modern generations to reconstruct almost the whole edifice of science." This was said about two generations ago and the rebuilding has only partly begun. It therefore makes little difference where one begins unless perchance it can be discovered where the modern prejudices against it are the weakest. I have not been able to discover this point of entry, and therefore I choose to jump with Daremberg and others in medias res, namely Galenic medicine, and since that is so pervasive in its influence in ancient medicine, I choose to enter at the centre, namely Galen's physiology and the centre of that, his teleology. I believe this is a better choice for a philosopher than, say, the many empirical points where Galen could be shown to be right, judged even by modern instrumental and empirical standards. The teleology is the well-known black mark that even those who have not read him know to be placed on his system. If one is to condemn him, this is certainly the point of easy attack. Likewise if one is to understand him and his physiological insights, this is the place from which to view the rest. Most of what I have to say has been worked out as I have read *On the Natural Faculties* and the *Utility of Parts*, although its consequences pervade all his writings.

It is difficult even for the inquiring reader to follow Galen's diffuse, verbose, meandering style with anything like a sympathetic comprehension. It cannot be true that he wrote all of his books when he was an old man, and yet that is the persistent impression they make on the modern reader. He admires Plato and Hippocrates to the point of quoting their writings as scriptures or as mystical wisdom books; he fights bitter controversies not only with his living contemporaries, but with dead predecessors; he makes speeches of exhortation and prayers of invocation before and after his analytical expositions of the parts of the body and their functions. There is so much of this kind of rhetoric in his works that one is tempted to use the scissors and paste ruthlessly in order to amputate and eliminate the sentimental ravings of a pious old dodo. But with time and patience the persistent reader comes to see that this would be a fatal mistake, the mistake that I fear has been made by almost all modern readers, for without scissors and paste they have managed to suppress or ignore the vital thread that runs through the discourse.

It should not be forgotten that Galen was heir to almost a thousand years of Greek thought and culture, and that he was bringing it all to bear on the professional problems of medicine. It is therefore necessary to catch his interpretation of Greek thought in order to keep his own work in focus. I believe this can best be stated in

terms of the doctrine of signatures as that enters and
enriches the Greek concern with the theory and practice
of the arts.   Galen's writings are thus a medical interpretation of Greek life and thought, and have a great
deal to do with the tradition of humanism in all subsequent
European thought.

It will be recalled that the doctrine of signatures sees
man as a somewhat tender delicate creature dependent
on the rest of the world and subject to its favouring or
destructive powers.   Human life is precarious, and in its
early or primitive stages is always short, brutish, and
nasty.   Security, success, and happiness are only to be
achieved by the discovery of the ways and means of life
and their isolation, regulation, and refinements.   God, or
the gods, have created ways and means sufficient to the
needs of life, but they are hidden and only half formed
for man's immediate use.   According to Espinas in *Les
Origines de la Technologie* there were two Greek tempera-
ments and two schools of thought regarding the mode of
discovery and cultivation of the ways and means.   One
held that the gods revealed to man the instruments and
the rules for turning them to their uses.   The gods also
imposed disciplines upon men, and commanded them to
conform to the corresponding institutions and customs.
This view was quite unanimously held in the early years
of the Greek epoch.   The other view which began fairly
early but only gained predominance at the end was that
man had been endowed with powers and inclinations
through which he could discover for himself the ways and
means to his livelihood and happiness.   These views
refer, of course, to the divine institution and the human

invention of the arts, and have their counterparts even now in the naturalistic anthropological issue concerning the diffusion and invention of culture patterns. Espinas, who was himself a philosophical anthropologist, tells the outline story of Greek technical, social, and political history in terms of the struggle between these two views and the modes of life that correspond to them.

Galen had a somewhat subtler and better furnished mind than Espinas, and consequently manages to keep these views balanced in his analysis and in his use of the Greek notion of the arts. I believe it is this notion which provides at least one of the threads binding his medical thought into a system which dominated the theory and practice of medicine for the following fifteen centuries. He not only applied the notion to the medical arts themselves, but the notion of art becomes the regulative and the constitutive principle in the medical sciences. Needless to say, the notion of art which could carry this burden was not narrowly conceived ; it included the useful arts, the liberal arts, and the fine arts in all their variety and mutual connections.

A great many of the pious rhetorical passages which the impulsive scissors-and-paste editor would wish to eliminate from the Galenic texts are concerned with the admirable artistry of God in His creation of the human body, and the consequent and equally admirable artistry of the human body in its operations. These passages are usually understood as the sentimental religious expression of a wonder which is now currently expressed in the aphorism, Ain't Nature Grand. The two expressions have a lyrical connection, of course, but there is a great difference in them if they are thrown against their respective intellectual backgrounds. The modern expression is an expression of ignorance, or at most a challenge to empirical investigation. With Galen it is the expression of an enthusiasm for a biological principle which has a vast array of empirical exemplifications, a high heuristic value in the biological sciences, and a basic position in the rational sciences that constitute medical knowledge. The principle states that every part of the body has a use, a fitness, and an operation with an almost inexhaustible set of consequent utilities both within and outside the body itself.

This is usually taken to mean that Galen, or any teleologist that talks this way, is imputing anthropomorphic purposes, foreknowings, and powers of rational direction to sub-rational entities, and it is compared to the anthropologist's account of primitive animism according to which the savage projects his own feelings, wishes, and fears into the opaque and unintelligible things around him. I have my doubts about the projection that the anthropologist himself indulges in these accounts, but I have no doubts about Galen. His teleological accounts of the human body are based on a wider context of thought than his own or any other persons' wishes and fears, although these do find their subordinate places in his system. Greek thought cut through its sophistications about primitive animisms and projections, and by Galen's time has found a rational account of these phenomena and also of the guesswork of the sophists who supplied them with their anthropology.

Galen's account rests upon the analysis and application

of the notion of an art and his physiology arises from this source. Putting it flatly, Galenic physiology is the science that originated in the metaphor : The body is an artist. I do not know who first proposed the metaphor, but there is no doubt that it was an object of fascination, and as time went on of great practical and theoretical concern with the Greeks. By Galen's time its contexts had been explored continually from the time of the Sophists ; its content had been expanded into elements that could be exhibited since the time of Socrates and Plato ; and it had received a classical formulation in the writings of Aristotle. In fact it had served as matrix for many sciences besides physiology. Of course there were many other mythical and poetic sources from which science had arisen, but none more important and illuminating for a modern who needs to realize the width and depth of the gap he must bridge if he wishes to pass from modern to ancient understandings.

Probably the first and certainly the most persistent assumption that was made for the purpose of understanding the metaphor was that art is an imitation of nature, or the artist imitates nature. At first this is an unsophisticated remark, merely pointing out that art brings about changes that are similar to those in nature, but it is soon realized that the imitation itself introduces artifices that are not immediately recognized as like the ways of nature. The imitations of imitations that occur in a social group where one person, say an apprentice, copies the work of a master or inventor tend to throw the artifices into the foreground, and as habit becomes custom the artifice takes to itself an authoritative privilege. If this is questioned and really needs defence, the master will find an apology. If he is not an anthropologist or an historian of the technologies and folkways, he will take recourse to the notion of divine fabrication and extend the apprentice system to the gods. He himself will be the imitator of the gods. Thus the novelty introduced by the invention will have been a revelation, and he himself will become at least to his imitators a demigod who keeps divine company. Thus there were the legends of Prometheus and Epimetheus, Athena and Haphaestus, Aesclepius and Hippocrates.

As inventions multiply and the experience of initiating novelties increases there will be anthropologists and historians who will realize that the master has invented his apology also, and it will appear that man can generate his own folkways and techniques. The arts are then understood as human fabrications, and cleverness in observation and skill in manipulation will replace or at least modify the notion of imitation. It was this stage that was cultivated and formulated by the naturalistic and humanistic sophists.

But cleverness and skill will bear further investigation, and it was Socrates who noted that cleverness and skill taken by themselves do not explain the arts; they merely describe them. Without knowledge there is no excellence in the arts. Socrates spent his life trying to find out what this essential knowledge was and where it might be found, and as he did so the notion of imitation underwent its most remarkable change. The knowledge that guides imitation has a certain generality which seems to provide a foundation for regular recurrent applications.

The artist's practice is in some sense the transfer of forms from one material to another. But since nature shows continual change it cannot be the real source of the forms ; they seem to have an independent status. Imitation would then consist first in an observation of nature which itself seems to embody a form, second an abstraction and clarification of this form, and finally its introduction into a new material. This is a brief account of a rather long laborious preparation of the Greek mind for the distinction between form and matter. Socrates did not make it very clear and always seemed a bit dazed by its importance. It was obviously an important clue to the nature of the arts and itself was related closely to the current doctrine of ideas which had been cultivated and applied in the mathematical speculations of the followers of Pythagoras.

Plato's dialogues represent for us, as they did for Galen, an extended exploration of this distinction as it was applied to all sorts of arts, the useful, the intellectual, and the fine. The doctrine of ideas carried great prestige, partly because it was heir to the belief in divine fabrication, and partly because it maintained and progressively defined the fundamental distinction between form and matter. The practice of an art was the process by which forms were imitated and multiplied by man in material, and nature itself began to look like an artist whose works also participated in forms. The knowledge that had been seen to be essential in the arts turned out to be the knowledge of forms or ideas, and the doctrine of ideas with its eternities and necessities in logic became the proper subject-matter for the sciences of nature.

This discovery, recorded in the seventh book of the

Republic, is perhaps the most fateful turning point in the history of European thought. The knowledge embodied in and ruling the arts had up to that time been patronizingly called right opinion, a kind of workman's sense of fitness and propriety in thinking, not very far from the correctness of the incantations that go with magic. The critical examination of right opinion, begun by the sophists and culminating in Plato, split conventional workaday opinion into two parts, that which was accepted as guesswork or hearsay, and that which could be learned and taught, added to, and corrected by a new use of intelligence. There followed from this a distinction in the arts themselves between the useful and the liberal, and one may add a social distinction between the craftsman and the freeman. The distinction between the arts was not merely a distinction in the material means by which they were practised, but rather a distinction between the ends for which they were practised. The useful arts were practised for the obvious ends of changing and transforming things. The liberal arts were practised for the sake of knowledge or science. Science might have its pragmatic locus between the beginning and end of the change, and a pragmatic function of contributing to the organization of the means, but it was also immediately recognized that it had also a directive commanding position with respect to the useful arts. The ideas which it discovered and analysed also represented the values or goods that validated the ends. It is not mere chance that prompted Galen to write an essay exhorting medical students to the study of the liberal arts in which he makes the now famous remark that he who would be a physician must also be a philosopher. Philosophy was the name for the love of wisdom which laboriously brought explicit knowledge of forms into the human arts.

It would seem probable that Aristotle, a student under Plato in the Academy, which was founded to explore and survey ideas, would follow his master in the abstract development of the mathematics, logic, and metaphysics. This is apparently what happened as long as Aristotle was actually in the Academy, but as soon as he withdrew, he felt himself graduated from the discipline of the liberal arts and turned to the next stage of establishing and formulating the sciences which the findings of the liberal arts made possible. Although Plato had laid down the rules for both an ascending and descending dialectic among ideas, his own genius had performed its greatest feats in the direction of ascent, and consequently his greatest achievements were discoveries of ideal regions and vistas. The descending dialectic which would result in organization and consolidation of knowledge demanded the genius of an Aristotle. Another way of saying the same thing is this : Plato had found material things significant only as they raised intellectual difficulties ; he flew only after he had stumbled. Aristotle found material things necessary instruments and media for any consequential dealings with ideas. He also found them necessary as the occasions and principles for specification. Aristotle, like his famous student Alexander, found it a duty to conquer the world ; he thought it essential to lay the foundations of the arts in genuine scientific knowledge.

It is one of the marvels of history that Aristotle, the man who saw the possibility of doing this, also had the

ability to accomplish it. To a modern it is even more
surprising that he did his best scientific work on man
and living things, the subject-matter with which we are
the feeblest. The secret of his success, I believe, lies in
his nearness to the discovery of the arts and the consequent directness of his application of their findings.
He accepted the suggestion that lies in the less cultivated
side of Platonism, namely that nature is an artist, and he
immediately accepted the consequences of this for the
arts themselves. The artist imitates nature because
nature is the supreme artist. This at once takes account
of the material that nature provides and lays nature open
to endless exploration and organization. It is in this
context that the Aristotelian terminology becomes
intelligible, as it was for Galen.

It is often said in adverse criticism of Aristotle, that,
being heir to a great literary tradition, he read literature
into nature, that he, in short, made nature a literary
artist. If that were literally true it would mean that
Aristotle achieved a far greater success than he actually
did, and the criticism would be thought adverse only by
him who is unaware of the pervasive and permanent
influence of the literary tradition in modern science. As
a matter of fact Aristotle's analysis of nature in terms of
the arts is also an analysis of the arts as parts of nature.
The terms artificial and natural become convertible as
the analysis shows the way for rendering all things
rational, and this is the end toward which all science
works.

The first step in the rationalizing of an art is to relativize
the distinction between form and matter. Since all things

are seen to be matter in some form, or formed matter, the fact that art changes things means that a material that has one form can become with its form the matter for a still other form, and since the result is again formed matter it can again receive another form, etc. So that the distinction between form and matter which has sharp and definite application in any given art, will have a relative and moving application in the series of arts that change matter from one thing to another progressively. Accordingly, on the theoretical side, science which is primarily concerned with the abstraction of forms will make distinctions between form and matter that are respectively relative to the specific constituent arts within comprehensive arts.

Consequently, in the transformations that art brings about, the forms that have already been introduced into material will determine the capacity of the things to receive additional forms. Thus if we say that material has the general potentiality to receive forms, it will follow that forms already received determine specific potencies. This serves to show the inter-relations between the Aristotelian terms form and matter, and potency and act, the last being the term that applies to the reception and maintenance of a form by matter. This is an account of the passive mode of the artistic process.

The active mode of the artistic process involves another set of terms which are badly understood in Aristotle without the nature-artist metaphor. The changes that are brought about by artistic transformation are due to agents, grossly represented in the archetypal case by the artist himself. A finer analysis shows that the artist is a complex entity divisible into a source of movement, or first mover, and various kinds of moved movers, or mediums for communicating change. On further analysis it appears that the first mover is infinitely removed, in fact belongs to another order of being, and that the artist as proximate agent is merely a moved mover. But the artist also has directive powers, or active potencies, and these are closely related to the formal content of the relevant science.

The directive powers are forms dictating the ordering of means to the end for which the art is practised, and they are formulated in the rules of the art. This is the artistic context for the famous four causes which go into any transformation, whether natural or artificial. There are the material causes representing the passive material that is to undergo transformation; the formal cause found in the knowledge of the artist, in the rules of practice, or in the laws of the change; the efficient causes, formed matters that act as moved movers; and the final cause or end product for which the art is practised.

The Platonic emphasis on form in the arts and the distinction between form and matter have here been re-interpreted to apply to natural change. Potency and act correspond to the distinction between form and matter but in such a way that the machinery of causation has been introduced at the same time. This is one of the revisions that Plato would have gladly accepted, but would not have taken the trouble to formulate; it provides a descending dialectic by which the understandings vouchsafed by ideas take on the responsibilities of natural science. The result is a science of physics.

But this is not all of physics. The strictures placed on a rational account of change by Parmenides and Zeno and formulated in the famous Paradoxes of Zeno forced Aristotle to a closer examination of the rationale of change. His solution of the paradoxes, which had arisen from a vague conception of matter taking on successive forms, can again be stated in term of the arts. Matter which is now little more than the name for the capacity to take on forms exists as an ordered set of potencies of a sub-stratum or substance, and change is the realization of these potencies which inhere in the substance. The potencies when actualized are acts of the substances which are, as it were, natural artists co-operating, supplement-ing, guiding, and sometimes teaching the human artist. In fact both the human artist and the natural artist are substances with potencies to be realized in their proper co-operative acts. Galenic medicine is an elaboration of this last Aristotelian point, but there are other Aristotelian points that we must note before we pass on to the medical application.

In addition to this substantial and dynamic machinery the sciences which Aristotle aimed to build needed a machinery of classification as it is usually called. It is true that the predicaments and predicables which arise from his analysis of propositions as they occur in science give rise to classes and classifications, but again the real upshot of his doctrine was a matrix of terms for the formulation of the routes of change which artistic pro-cesses followed. Observed natural changes do not at first sight seem to follow definite routes, at least not routes that correspond with artistic and rational rules.

In other words substances have accidents as well as properties, accidents when they do not obey rules, properties when they do. Properties, moreover, are related according to rules and laws, which can be stated in propositions of general import and are subject to the rules of logic. Furthermore, the terms in the propositions, the genera and species, fall into mutually exclusive categories according to their modes of predication in propositions. The complex relations of inclusion and exclusion in this categorical hierarchy determine possible routes for change, and the successive substitution of predicates in propositions according to the rules of the syllogism gives rise to systems of propositions that rationally describe natural changes. The art of rational discourse imitates nature, and its product is science.

These, in the briefest outline that I can make, are the doctrines that are set forth in the *Organon, Physics, and Metaphysics* of Aristotle. For two thousand years they were the working intellectual equipment of all learned and technical work in Europe, Asia Minor, and northern Africa. Even on the obvious pragmatic level of criticism this means that Aristotle's formulation of the sciences and their foundations had a direct relevance to the arts as they were practised, and it is hardly a wise judgment that condemns it for having diverted scientific thought from a line that only in the last two or three hundred years has been judged to be right. Still this has to be explained.

There is the obvious and oft repeated comment that the clarity and comprehensiveness of the Aristotelian formulation is a danger in itself. The work of science is made so easy by such formulation that it can be done only by stupid people. The best minds will turn to the unformulated. Clarity breeds contempt. But these are external remarks evidencing ignorance of the content of the Aristotelian statements. It is again only a superficial mind that finds Aristotle's clarity easy to achieve. The genuine explanation is to be derived from the peculiarities of the disagreements between Plato and Aristotle, and these disagreements appear most strikingly in their interpretations of mathematics. Curiously enough these interpretations are not incompatible ; they are merely divergent and complementary, and should not have had the profound and persistent splitting effect on the history of thought that they seem to have had.

The Greek experience with mathematics started very early and was continuous throughout a period of about a thousand years. As we understand this period its mathematical thought appears as a kind of obligato parallelling at a distance and echoing in varying degrees of harmony the main line of development in the useful and liberal arts. There are apparently two or three occasions when it is to be identified with this main line. In order to understand this rather striking independence we must take note of certain peculiarities in the practice of the mathematical arts. It is customary to look for an empirical and practical origin for them, especially in Egyptian land surveying, and there is a certain neat plausibility about this account. But it does not take account of peculiarities intrinsic to mathematics itself that are at least as relevant as its empirical applications. It seems that mathematics has always had a touch of divine madness in its aim and method, or if you like, a certain artificiality in its manner. It seems probable that the first scientific instruments, such as the surveying ropes and the balance, were invented by mathematicians who saw the need of artificial constructions for precision and stability in practice. But on the whole it seems that the makers of the instruments followed the example of the makers of language and seized upon more easily manipulable things which they could arbitrarily transform and apply generally over wide ranges of things. Ropes and levers are, of course, such things, but the letters of the alphabet are still better since they can be made with little effort by the human tongue or the pen. Out of ropes, levers, tongues, and pens, come the compass and the graduated ruler with arithmetic and geometry as obvious results.

The peculiarity of the arts for which these provide the instruments is their artificiality in the vulgar sense and their apparent freedom from the usual restraints that nature imposes on the other arts. The only comparably independent arts are literary, and these only when they approach the state of pure poetry. Therefore, ingenuity and invention will be at their peak in the mathematical arts and the mathematician will easily feel himself inspired and think of his products as oracular in character. His products may reach high degrees of elaborateness before he finds occasion or inclination to apply them or find them in nature. This is, of course, what happened in the Pythagorean development, and it is not surprising that an esoteric religious cult immediately arose. For the ordinary person mathematics has always been crypto-grammatic and not a little mysterious, and there has been fear and suspicion among the uninitiated corresponding to the distance between the esoteric and exoteric under-standings thus set up. The expert who dares cross the line between will be thought a magician, and will suffer persecution as demon-possessed or adulation as a priest as he fails or succeeds in gaining prestige. Mathematics does not diffuse its skills and ideas as easily as many of the other more familiar arts do.

On the other hand, the expert who succeeds in gaining prestige and can show results in the concrete applications of mathematics may easily be overwhelmed by the power that has been thrust upon him. Some such success met Democritus. I do not know just what feats of engineering got him his influence, but it seems very probable that he very early turned back from such exploitation of his knowledge and plunged his energies into something very like modern laboratory investigations, and as a result came out with a theory of the world which bears the marks of keen observation as well as extraordinary mathematical powers. The theory of material atoms with which he and Leucippus are credited is the simplest and most impressive example of what happens when nature is credited with the skills, rules, and precisions of a sophisticated human art. Pythagoras had allowed numbers to behave as presiding deities over natural processes, but Democritus put numbers into nature, and made her an exclusively mathematical genius. The atoms have none but mathematical properties, save possibly their innate motion which imitates the operations of translation and rotation invented by the mathematician for his ruler and compass. Furthermore, the atoms do not have to be very well educated in mathematics. The most elementary arithmetic and geometry will suffice to guide them and save the appearances ; bare quantity will be the highest mathematical conception that needs to be embodied. Democritus's atoms as things are almost as exoteric as Pythagoras's beans were, but they serve the immediate scientific purpose, and mathematics for once gets into the other arts by aiding the engineer. The results have never been wholly forgotten, and when they were put to new tasks in the seventeenth century, accelerated both scientific thought and the practice of the useful arts as they never had been accelerated before.

Instrumental techniques never caught up with the possibilities in Greek atomic theory, and when the attempt was made to further educate the atoms in mathematics, it was the Pythagorean Plato who disembodied the atoms and they ended as merely hypothetical entities with a tendency to a purely formal status. Plato's atoms were more than quantities and therefore receded to the Pythagorean esoteric position in the thought of the Greeks. The Academy cultivated a mathematical idealism, developed a calculus of proportions, systematized the discoveries already made, and passed on the results to the Alexandrians, one of whom, Euclid, formulated them in his *Elements*. This ideal development teased and tormented Greek thought from the first to the last, and we find its response in certain terms which it borrowed from this wayward art. Measure, symmetry, harmony

means between extremes, number as applied to poetry—
these are the vague traces of the divine science left in
all sorts of materials and activities.

Aristotle tried to incorporate mathematics within his
naturalization of the arts, but in spite of the validity of
his interpretations never managed to clip its speculative
wings without killing its vital centre. For him mathematics was an attributive science and its terms were
merely derivative. The consequent restrictions were
never accepted by the original mathematician. The
argument reaches its height in the discussions of infinity,
a term dear to the mathematician's heart and necessary
to his art and science, but never amenable to alien
subordination without loss of content. On the other
hand, Aristotle's criticism of mathematics does bring it
into the integral pattern of the arts and gives it a workable
place in nature. Nature is a mathematical artist but she
takes her mathematics with her other skills and duties in
a sober manner.

The development of the sciences following the fundamental work of Aristotle shows the split in the great
tradition. This is marked by sharp controversy between
the mathematicians and the logicians whenever a new
step is taken, and since both sides of the controversies
usually have a metaphysical as well as a technical interest,
each point of view achieves an ever increasing clarity and
power in first rate minds. In second rate minds there are
the intellectual monstrosities that compromise breeds.
No one seems to have achieved the bifocal insight which
would compose the actually complementary differences,
although there are near approaches to such insight in

many of the attempts at compromise. One side argues continually that the sciences tend in their maturity toward mathematics; the other side argues that each science sets up its own particular method and finds its own subject-matter, and that mathematics in particular is only one among many sciences, with logic alone as the universal instrument or organon. We at present are witnessing the latest battle between arts, and the mathematicians seem to be having the better of it. Galen is an interesting victim of the split. He seems to admire Plato more than Aristotle, but his method and results are almost purely Aristotelian. By sacrificing the bifocal insight and facing the problems of physiology I believe he is right. The controversy is, after all, only a fight between the artists, who are protecting the integrities of their respective arts. The problem remains unsolved to this day although the solution is taken for granted every time anything is measured.

In spite of such unsolved problems there is a certain completeness in the Greek exploration and analysis of the arts, and the results have become the European heritage of science. This is so profoundly true that in spite of the dark and middle ages and the attempts to circumvent them by renaissance, reformation and revolution, Europeans have continually rediscovered that it is impossible to step outside of the tradition. We must select and advance within the all-embracing set of assumptions that the Greeks made.

They practised and theorized the arts until the notion of art itself was generalized and rationalized to such a degree that it was possible to recognize art in man, art in nature, and art in divinity. Science being the detection of artifice was an inevitable consequence of the recognitions, and the intellectual imperative to discover the artifice in each art led immediately to the establishment of corresponding sciences. The result is a hierarchy of arts and a parallel hierarchy of sciences.

CHAPTER VI

THE HUMAN BODY AS ARTIST

I WOULD remind the reader again of the difficulties encountered by the modern mind attempting to bring this ancient lore into the context of scientific discourse. Patience is necessary not only in following the present exposition, but also in withholding adverse judgment of the doctrine whose familiarity in commonsense discourse has bred so much scientific contempt. It is said that the doctrine is sheer anthropomorphism, the ogre that dogs scientific progress at every step. I think that we shall find the ogre a spirit of light if we turn and face it at this point. In less dramatic language anthropomorphism is a constant inescapable phase of all science, and it is only by explicit recognition and rationalization that we can hope to divest ourselves of the illusion that we are free from it.

There are several senses in which science may be called anthropomorphic. In one sense it may be said that science is imputing human habits to inhuman or inanimate nature, and thus falsifying what is essentially neutral. It seems that the Greeks in the account just preceding were committing this pathetic fallacy in a shameless grand style. Nature is an artist ; how could the fallacy be more directly and comprehensively stated ? Or again it may be said that science is the verbal and symbolic expression of the nature of things, and in so far as the notations or symbols are artificial and conventional inventions they give a human twist to the truth and thus distort its unconventional purity. Finally, pursuit of science arises primarily from a boyish or apish curiosity, and the announcement of discoveries and secrets explained smacks too obviously of the many boastful and smart tricks by which we all too human beings deceive ourselves. Current as well as ancient science must plead guilty of all these charges, and much of the acrimony of current controversy is due to a feeling of guilt which is passed on to colleagues, predecessors, and finally to Aristotle himself, instead of being responsibly admitted.

There is still another sense in which science, particularly medical science, may be said to be anthropomorphic. In some sense human beings are always the subject-matter of science. Latter-day philosophic discussion of scientific method and epistemology repeatedly expresses one common article of faith, that the data of science are human sensations, the human effects of external causes, the results of human observation, the products of human manipulation. In the medical sciences, anatomy, physiology, and pathology, it is inescapable that the human body, which these sciences cannot completely reduce to chemical, physical, or biological materials without losing status, not only contributes but on the observable level wholly provides the subject-matter. The ubiquity of the human body is the source and the explanation for all the other grades and varieties of anthropomorphism. Man in relation to many other things is the inescapable and all-pervasive proper study of man. All the natural sciences are primarily medical in their origin and intent, as the myth of signatures suggests, and we shall be doing a service not only to medicine but to all the natural sciences if we make Galen speak again of the sciences that men study, the sciences that study men in the context of the arts that men practice.   This is radical and unreserved anthropomorphism, and it is the Galenic medical man who will face his obligation to follow out its consequences, and reformulate that hard-headed humanism which is so indispensable not only for culture in general but for science itself.

When in the fairly recent history of European culture the financial arts had become important enough to draw the attention of trained minds, there was developed an art of accounting within which there were the suggestions of a science of accounting.   In the course of time these suggestions blossomed into an elaborate set of economic sciences among which was double-entry book-keeping.   It is no wonder that catastrophes like the great depression have been blamed on the vicious abstraction and specula- tive irresponsibility of the certified accountant who professes this art and science.   Into his ledger there go symbols which distinguish between creditor and debtor when only one man is involved.   One and the same item is entered twice in these subtle books, and the accounts are not approved unless one and the same sum appear on both sides of the ledger.   The duplicity here is worthy of the subtlest lawyer, and I believe is only matched by the devious ways of the legal profession in modern thought. There it is supposed that the lawyer learned his distinction- making from the theologian, who found three persons in one God. It will be no news to the medical man that his own predecessors multiplied entities beyond the limits set by modern scientific styles in economy of thought. It may be news that he is still dealing with the multiplied entities but has no insight into the system in which they once made sense. The tendency to drop any kind of multiple book-keeping in the natural sciences is understandable as the consequence of current empirical enthusiasms, but it lays a heavy burden on the auditor who is called in to certify the accounts, a burden that obviously is too heavy for the philosophers who have volunteered their services and a burden beyond the competence of the empirical scientist, such as Lloyd Morgan, who has devised the infinitely multiple-entry book-keeping of emergent evolution. Emergent evolution is really a device for putting off the day of final accounting indefinitely, just as the theory of the migration of organs uses the rubrics of Darwinian evolution to avoid the application of any rigorous system of accounting to the riddles of human anatomy.

The metaphysics of form and matter supplies a system of double-entry book-keeping for any science, and although a science such as chemistry or physics may dodge the necessity, it seems that medicine which is man's study of man should not take chances in its attempt to avoid the anthropomorphic tangles that such a study threatens to involve. It should construct a system which would meet the present multidimensions of its subsidiary sciences.

In the first place it should be noted that multiplication of entities is not an accurate description of the effects of Aristotelian doctrine in science. It is rather the opposite, the systematization of the entities that a supposedly single-entry science has produced, and the placing of entities in systematic connections. Previous to Plato and Aristotle the artist, his material, and his product were separate entities, and furthermore there was a sharp distinction between the artificial and the natural. The effect of the Platonic and Aristotelian dialectic was to define things in such a way that each one was a substance which was at the same time but still intelligibly and distinctly an artist, a material, and a product. At the first step in the dialectic it was recognized that everything had its appropriate form ; at the second step it was discovered that this meant that one and the same thing was both form and matter. This parallels the dialectic in the development of accounting where debtor and creditor were first identified with separate persons, and then found to exist in the same person. The economist has still to discover the right way of reminding himself that any member of a market is both producer and consumer.

The next step in the Aristotelian system of accounting was the introduction of another dual scheme that would give cross references, and this turned out to be the agent and the product, taken from the notion of the artist and his work. The result is a system of quadruple entry book-keeping in which one and the same thing appears as matter, form, agent and end-product, or material, formal, efficient, and final cause. It is, of course, possible to build a science in which one of these terms sets the route for thought to take and leaves the others implicit, but such a science, for instance, chemistry, would not be medicine. Inanimate or inhuman matter may suffer such partial treatments without protest, but the human body will burst out with the suppressed principles and characters. It will claim consideration for the organism as whole and in all its guises. If medical men pay exclusive attention to muscles and bones, they will be haunted by ghosts, and will thus pay for their subterfuges by considering the formal and final causes in their sleep.

Of course our language is still loose. The human body is a substance which has a great variety of accidents, which may be classified grossly as essential, proper, and accidental, and these accidents are further subdivided according to their places in the genus-species matrix, and they are ordered according to the artistic rules which things obey. Finally the things thus understood in their many guises are the self-moving things that constitute the system of nature.

The human body thus becomes a most marvellous work of natural art. It is an artist fabricating tissues, organs, fluids, and gases out of the raw materials which it manages to procure from subsidiary arts. On the other hand it is the product of its own art ; the body taken at any moment or over a period, is a most exhaustively worked or informed material. Form and matter are most intimately combined on many levels and in the smallest detail, and there is nothing in the body that can be called merely matter, nor yet pure form. The doctrine lends itself easily to Galenic rhetoric, but, as I have said before, Galenic rhetoric is not empty of theoretical content. Certain doctrines flow from the complicated insight so rhetorically expressed, and the proof of the oratory will be in the exposition of these doctrines.

First there is a consequence in the Galenic method, again a kind of double voiced exposition which we have come to call the deductive and inductive method of rational procedure. Each of Galen's points of doctrine is expounded twice in his book on physiology, *On the Natural Faculties*, and for good measure there are dialectical interludes. One exposition is deductive and from the point of view of demonstration might stand by itself. The second exposition is inductive or descriptive of observation, dissection, or experimentation. Here, again, the modern mind is bored with what seems unnecessary verbal repetition, and a perverted sense of elegance. Actually Galen is making his verbal behaviour keep faith with his scientific process of thought. An ancient scientist did not think himself intellectually dishonest if he had made explicit beforehand what he expected or rationally should demand of observation and experiment. In fact he would have thought himself merely a sophist if he regularly met nature with a blank mind and waited to be persuaded by her many uncriticized charms. The only safe way to meet fact was to be well supplied with ideas in good order ; the maximum order and even the maximum number of ideas can be handled only by logic. All else is elusive opinion. It is only because common sense has been through the discipline of ancient logic that we suppose we can dispense with *a priori* demonstration. Galen even wrote a book on logic in the orthodox Aristotelian style properly adjusted to the needs of medical science.

Galen's inductive procedures are again puzzling to the modern mind. For instance, there is no talk of Mill's methods, and very little generalizing from the particular. The inductive accounts are descriptions or rules for the arts of observation, dissection, and experimentation. Experimentation is perhaps the most illuminating illustration of the procedure. The idea suggested by the deductive theory is transferred to the medium of the material under inquiry, or even better to a material such as the body of an animal which is not directly under inquiry but particularly adapted for the special features relevant to the idea. It was Vesalius in the fifteenth century who rediscovered with great excitement that Galen's anatomy had been done on animals rather than on man ; Galen by animal dissection had been able to give inductive expositions of human anatomy which had carried the medical arts for over a thousand years. Vesalius continued the method in human anatomy. Experimentation for Galen was the application of practical reason to concrete materials ; it was an art by which ideas in his mind induced ideas in things, and deduction was completed by operations on materials. He is very angry with his predecessors who allowed speculative Democritean atomism to take the place of detailed observation and experiment, and reports his own experiments with directions for repetition in order to refute childish mechanical theories put forth earlier by Erisistratus. Induction is not a method of proof ; it is a check and fulfilment of deductive thought. In this he is bringing his own and his pupils' rational souls to bear upon the activities of the vegetative and animal souls of men and animals. This is the traditional canonical form of medical research, a consistent and powerful extension of the diagnostic art practised at the bedside.

In order to get at the next important doctrine, the doctrine of the natural faculties, we must return to the hierarchy of forms and their various incidences in matter. Prime matter has infinite potentiality; it has the possibility of taking on an infinity of forms. However, there is an order of incidence with appropriate degrees of freedom within it at every step of the informative process. The first form achieved by a given matter, determines to a definite degree what further forms can be added. There will be impossible forms, possible forms, and necessary forms consequent upon the first substantial form attained. Thus it is that forms determine potentiality, or in briefer words, forms are potencies, powers of action and passion or change. Thus what is a formal cause of a tissue, namely its specialized tissue-form, is at the same time a potency of the organ to which the tissue belongs, and the form of that organ again a power of the organism to which it in turn belongs.

The science of physiology then consists, in so far as it is the investigation of dynamic properties of organisms, in the discernment and rational formulation of potencies of the parts of the body. When they are discerned and formulated they are called faculties. Formulation of potencies builds a rational science within which deduction is a legitimate procedure, and observation of bodily processes in their varieties and modes clarifies and amplifies *a priori* theory.

But we are already treading soil that has been consecrated by many battles of words. Powers, potencies, faculties, and other occult entities come ultimately from Macedonia, and Demosthenes was more prophetic than he knew when he warned the Athenians of the Macedonian dangers. King Aristotle ruled a vast intellectual empire well for two thousand years, but at the end of that time as everybody knows Macedonia has been a Balkan state. It is well to remember two things as we penetrate this land of barbaric superstitution. The first is that the body is an artist and that the powers which Galen called faculties are artistic powers. The second thing to remember is that Aristotle and Galen ruled by dividing the items of observation and analysis according to the rules of a quadruple-entry system of accounting. On one side of the ledger are the capacities of the parts of the body to operate in specific ways ; by virtue of these powers the parts of the body are the artistic agents, or efficient causes. On another side of the ledger there are the elementary constituents of the body, earth, air, fire, and water, with their principles, the hot and the cold, the wet and the dry. These are relatively material causes in the artistic production. One can balance these two kinds of entry of items, for it is these materials with their minimum forms that determine the capacities of the agents in the process. A third entry can be distinguished in the higher forms governing directly the operations of the agents and through them the material constituents. These are the faculties which in Galenic physiology are usually attributed to the organs and the humours. Finally in the fourth column these same forms are integrated and entered as souls, the entelechies or actualities of the body. Again the two latter columns, forms and ends, balance if the observation and analysis has been sound, and finally the former columns with their balance between materials and agents balance with the latter pair and their balance, and we can say with some clarity and without intent to deceive that the soul is the well-balanced harmony of the body.

It should not be difficult to see this hierarchy of potencies and forms as levels of analysis and integration, and to realize that the accounts will eventually balance if they are not fudged. It is not so easy to see that a fourfold account has any advantages that compensate for the risks that such complication always involves. Galen's answer to that question if given to-day would be direct and up to date ; he would say that a fourfold accounting system is also a check on irresponsible speculation and would add that it is also a check on irresponsible observation. On the one hand, the material and efficient causes demand analytical observation and the anchoring of the theory in the discrete parts of the body ; on the other hand, the inquiry and formulation of the formal and final causes insures the clarity and consistency of the rational content of the science. It can hardly be hoped that these two large divisions will advance *pari passu* or with smooth agreement. There must be times when the physiological budget must go unbalanced, but the explicit scheme for balancing will act as a constant reminder of scientific obligations. Galen's own physiological theory and his very elaborate anatomy were not always in agreement, notably in the case of the pores in the septum of the heart which he theoretically demanded but admitted he had never observed. It is interesting to note here that it was observation dictated by a theory taken from Aristotle that enabled Harvey to revise the Galenic theory of the circulation of the blood.

With regard to the controversy over the occult entities that reached its height during the Renaissance this can be said. Late medieval Galenists named the faculties in the organs according to the theory of forms and matter. They then reified them as bodies and inserted them in the organs. Their double book-keeping had slipped a column and then had materialized all the columns, so that one looked for corporeal fairies and hobgoblins in the brain, behind the liver, and above the heart, and the rational immortal soul was expected to spread its wings on the death of the body and soar to the stars. They not only multiplied entities, they duplicated and quadrupled bodies, much as the keepers of the gold reserve would do if they completely lost functional insight and control of the commercial world. The name for such entities should not be occult ; they are all too obvious. They were the creations of imaginations whose intellectual light had slipped into the lower phase of corporeal matter, and the result was a Balkanized science, and Europe was quite right in its intolerance. This is the constant danger of systems of book-keeping, and the better the system the more numerous and probable are the degradations. The dominance of the mechanical style of explanation and the reliance on bacteriology as the basis for contemporary pathological theory is an extension of the same imaginative ingenuity to our own time. The one human body is multiplied and distributed without benefit of certified accountants. It would seem that single-entry book-keeping also has its devices for the mass production of entities. Galenic theory finds one body enough and turns to abstract thought for its distinctions and the enrichment of its insights ; Galen sometimes suggests that not four but five causes should be found if the artistic operations under inquiry show that much subtlety.

The book *On the Natural Faculties* applies this machinery to the analytical exposition of the nutritive arts of the body. These are the arts over which the vegetative soul presides, but he says at the outset that he personally would prefer not to call these faculties souls. Apparently he already, even in Alexandria, felt the dangers of too much talk about the soul, although he says he does not object if his readers understand what he has to say in those terms.

In this account the body is understood as the artist fabricating itself, and the various internal organs, mouth, stomach, intestines, liver, heart, and spleen, are engaged in specialized subsidiary arts that contribute to the total making. Galen is tireless and acrimonious in discrediting his predecessor, Aesclepiades, who thought that his ingenuity in mechanical speculation relieved him of the necessity to dissect and observe the mechanisms that they imputed to the body. Galen defends the body from such slander of its admirable artistry. I am reminded of the modern faith in the circulation of the blood which has left it unexplained to the present how the venous blood returns to the heart when the hydrostatic pressure in the veins of the leg is never equal to the demands of the observed facts, and this in turn reminds one of the acceptance of Harvey's theory of circulation before the observation of the capillary circulation.   Harvey merely speculatively moved the pores in the heart to the arteries and veins.   In Galen's day the problem was a simpler one of how the urine went from the kidneys to the bladder, and we should credit him with the insistence against the mechanists that the already observed duct had something to do with it.

Galen is also tireless and rigorous in his inference from the generic nature of processes like genesis, growth, and nutrition to the specific processes of bodily fabrication. The nature of these fabrications is stated in terms of Aristotle's *Physics*, which, with Plato's *Timaeus*, is always the source of Galen's first premises.   These premises are concerned with the formal and final causes for which Aristotle and Plato supply the proper deductive machinery. As can be seen genesis, growth, and nutrition, are cases of the three pairs of kinds of change, generation and corruption, increase and decrease, assimilation and differentiation, respectively.   At the other end of the process of fabrication there are the nutriments which are various mixtures of the four elements.   The body as artist has to find the raw material of nutriment, procure, prepare, attract, select, present, and assimilate it, according to the distinct yet related potencies of both passive external material and active internal faculty.

Cooking and diet are always in the back of the Greek medical man's mind.   Beginning with the Hippocratic writing *On Ancient Medicine* there are treatises which give the history of medicine as a development out of the arts of cooking.   In Aristotle we find that the nearest he came to an account of chemical processes was when he distinguished between the various kinds of cooking, with fire as usual the medium for the application of the principle of heat.   Galen is full of analogies with pumps and such suggestive devices, but the allegory within which all of them fit is the analogy which would see the body as a self-cooker.   The principle of attraction is the form that governs the local motion involved in nutrition from the distribution of the nutriment to the selection of it by the proper organs, tissues, and humours.   Each organ does its specific sort of cooking according to the forms which determine its capacities or potencies and appropriates or passes on the product according to its powers of selection and assimilation.   Alteration of qualities is the physical principle which is further analysed and applied in the final account of assimilation.

Quite apart from the analytical detail of this physiology, I see in it a very pretty application and elaboration of the doctrine of signatures.   In its application to man and the universe it has an epic grandeur, but it also shows itself capable of a very subtle and refined development reaching and penetrating to the finest distinctions and smallest minutiae of biological science.   It is not only man as a whole that has given to him the arts by which he can find and bend the rest of nature to his own ends ; it is the same capacity that has been given to each part, organ, or tissue, and, as we would say now, to each cell. Aristotle's *Physics* analyses the arts in such a versatile way that all varieties of natural activity and change can be brought under a single rational control.   That is important for science ; but it is doubly important for biological science in that it analyses without doing violence to the specifically biological and physiological activities of organisms. The problem of constructing a modern physics that will serve the same medical scientific ends will be treated later, but it should be noted here where it is most obviously important. Galen's rhetoric on the artistry of nature has, I believe, this philosophical and medical bearing.

So far I have been using Plato, Aristotle, and Galen as authoritative expositors of the central theme of the rationalistic tradition in science, namely the doctrine of forms. This doctrine does for the theoretical side what the doctrine of signatures does for the empirical side of science. The doctrine of signatures assumes that the data of science are potential symbols, and calls on the liberal arts and sciences to develop, clarify, and realize the potentialities of human observation. The practice of these arts and sciences ends in the discovery and formulation of abstract forms, and it is by reference to these forms that the data achieve their status as facts and scientific evidence.

The doctrine of forms takes up the scientific theme at this point. Forms are not only what signatures signify ; they are also the causes of things. They are therefore the proximate subject-matter of science. Plato makes the first extensive statement of the doctrine, and with him it is the insight of insights. Aristotle makes distinctions within the general doctrine and sets up a system of quadruple entry book-keeping for causes which is based on the fact that forms maintain themselves both in nature and in discursive science in a hierarchical order. The discernment of form which is the aim of science demands the concomitant distinction of at least three forms in the hierarchical order ; these in their proper sub- and super-ordination are the three causes, material, efficient, and formal. The fourth cause is the substantial being which results from the integration of these three forms with their appropriate matters. The essence of the thing as well as the substantial content of science is the formal cause through which the hierarchical integration takes place.

Just as the abstract form, when it is discovered and formulated in trivial logic, fixes and reifies the concrete data in their proper symbolic relations as fact and evidence, so the formal cause in natural science trans-figures and galvanizes the flux of natural change in a deterministic order governed by principle. Through forms signatures finally signify real causes.

The analogy that I have suggested here between the trivial arts and sciences and the natural arts and sciences is only an analogy ; that is, the things though compared actually lie in different metaphysical regions. But on the methodological level the analogy carries the burden of scientific analysis and it can be carried out in detail. Notations are the material causes in the trivial arts ; the rhetorical use of symbols in discourse parallels the manifold routes by which efficient causes act in nature ; and the general propositions of a science formulate formal causes. Diagnosis, and prognosis as well as therapy, imitate the causal order in the human body. Galen's faculties are forms between the soul and the natural elements, and they act in material and efficient ways according to their places in the hierarchy of forms.

We have finally come to the scientific Armageddon

which I have postponed to the end of the story, not
because ends come last in nature, but because they are in
some sense those things intelligible in themselves which
Aristotle says we arrive at last in the order of understanding. Teleology is for Galen the first principle of
natural science, and I am sure that he would with Plato
find it most clearly at work at present in mathematics
under other names. On the other hand, I do not think
he would understand how modern controversies over
teleology could be so awkwardly stated and met. He
would, of course, be horrified at his late medieval followers
who pounced with single-minded if not simple-minded
theological zeal on one of his most rhetorical teleological
words, πρόνους, foreknowledge. Taken from its theological context in the doctrine of God's providential
government of the world, applied first to man where such
flattery would have the worst consequences, and then lent
by Franciscan charity as it were to the animals and
plants, it confused theology and teleology profoundly and
perhaps permanently. The halls of academic philosophy
still reverberate with the thunder of the religious rhetoric
that followed. Then when the Reformation deformed
theology into ethics and ethics persistently degraded itself
to a more or less rational psychology and finally to an
empirical physics of man, the term good became a
by-word for all that is whimsical and wayward in human
will and appetite, and their objects. Under these
circumstances it was a waste of breath to say that the
good was not a scientific term, and it is no wonder that
we now read the famous passage in the *Republic* in which
Plato gravely says that the good is the principle of both

existence and value with a supercilious smile ; and further that we read all of Galen with a belletristic antiquarian interest.   Suffice it to say that I am not taking sides in the modern battle of the vitalists and the mechanists, neither of whom evidence an insight into entelechies, final causes, nor even vital principles.

The principle of teleology in its classical expressions and applications is none other than the principle of causal determinism explicated and stated in its fullness.   Fore-knowledge, on the other hand, is a term that appealed to the egotism of the early modern scientist who was taking the place of the astrologer and alchemist in his social functions.   It is in evidence still in the rhetorical use of the term prediction in the forensic science of the British and American Associations for the Advancement of Science.   Otherwise it is only the name for a bit of clever extrapolation done in the course of a laboratory experi-ment or at the hospital bedside.   It can be applied to man to say nothing of animals only as an expression of scientific wonder at the orderliness of events in nature as they appear in historical retrospect.

Similarly the quaint sounding phrase that everything happens for the sake of the good is in its context only a translation of the phrase that nature is orderly throughout. In the classical tradition good is a transcendental predicate and therefore predicable of everything, and its Aristotelian exegesis is that the matter in nature has found its appro-priate form or hierarchy of forms, and has thus realized its ends, at least partially.   To deny teleology in this sense would be not only to assert chaos but to attempt nonsense.

However, determinism and therefore teleology are not problems for empirical testing, except to find out which end and which means or matter are conjoined. They are, like the conservation of energy, general postulates ; in fact they are even more general postulates than the conservation of energy which is to be subsumed under them. Determinism merely makes it explicit that the essence of science is rationality and lays down a rule that things shall not be accepted as understood until they appear in a rational system. Teleology is the key stone in the arch of any rational science, and the science that ignores or denies it is merely announcing its present immaturity or its pig-headed irrationality.

Bergson made a clever point when he said that teleology is merely inverted mechanism, though I believe he missed the main point of his remark in his restriction of its significance to the inversion of mechanical action in the time series. Mechanism and teleology are reciprocals of each other, it is true, but the inversion and reciprocation are matters of double-entry book-keeping. As I have said, the columns in Aristotelian accounting represent levels of form and matter. If science is good the columns balance. What one sees as mechanism can also by a shift of attention or intention be seen as teleology. This is an elementary point in the doctrine of the four causes, and sets a standard by which much modern science is to be condemned.

This last point brings us back to the main import of Galenic science. It demands a thorough going mechanism and teleology, hence an exhaustive and explicit determinism in physiology. There is literally nothing in the organism, organ, tissue, cell, or body fluid which is to be eliminated as vestigial, supernumerary, functionless, or irrational. To be sure there are things in the body at any given stage of physiology which we do not understand, but the art is long, and the science is long enough to promise that it will, sooner or later, rationalize the as-yet-unrationalized. If it did not make that promise it could not be trusted to keep its aim rational, or scientific even in the modern sense. Determinisms are of many kinds and the present variety and versatility of scientific speculation promise well that teleology will come back into science, though perhaps shamefacedly and under disguise.

Recent controversy over determinism and the freedom of the will is hardly worth consideration here. I intend to be discussing principles rather than crises in science, but there is one aspect of it that may add a ray of light on the present darkness that hides the principle of determinism. The point is this : that determinism is a postulate of science and it states what the main character of the ideas in science shall be. To say that science has discovered indeterminism is therefore to say that science has discovered something about itself. This might mean that it had discovered an ultimate limitation, but if I understand the situation in sub-atomic physics it has rather discovered a possible avenue of extension which it has not yet seen the way to exploit. In Aristotelian terms science has discovered a lower order of matter and a higher order of forms which have not yet reached clear and adequate formulation. It means that the physicist knows something in a way that does not yet belong to physics, and we can hope that he will improve his knowledge rather than allow himself to fall too precipitately into superficial mysticism.

In general it should be remembered that free will is not incompatible with rationality, determinism, and teleology. All of these are principles of principles, that is to say, criteria regulating science. Science deals with abstractions and allows variability within the ranges of its abstractions; in fact its generality demands internal variability. A science formulates a hierarchy of laws and at the same time a gradation of freedoms, degrees of freedom, as they are called in mathematics and physics. All necessities hold within themselves the appropriate hypothetical liberties, ranges of existence and action that are consistent with themselves.

This allows the defence of a central Galenic point without taking sides with either the mechanistic or the theological determinist. The universality and exhaustiveness of teleological determinism leads to the metaphysical notion of the soul as the watchful and guiding form of the individual body. Galen prefers to speak only of the rational form of the body as the soul, and relegates the vegetable and animal souls of the Greek tradition to the category of natural faculties, but whatever the terminological preferences may be, it is clear that he is following his determinism to its logical conclusion, which, with the admission that human knowledge is always incomplete, would allow him to say with Scotus Erigena, we know that there is a soul, but we do not know what it is, or with other medievals, that we know what the soul is like, to wit, the form of an organ, but we do not know just what it is in the individual body. It is in this context with one eye on metaphysics and the other on the future of medicine, that we can say that the soul is the proper subject-matter of the medical sciences, and that all present medical science is without knowing it studying the human soul. But lest I try the patience of the modern reader too much, I hasten to expand this conclusion into a dialectical pattern through which free thought may escape the apparently dogmatic trap. The proposition that the soul exists is a metaphysical proposition, and this means that although it is an inescapable inference from the ordinary physiological statements, it is, like the geometrical statement that parallel lines meet at infinity, a statement of boundary conditions for the strictly scientific subject-matter. The soul is the paradoxical meeting point for the abstractions of science and the concrete individual units of nature ; it is the ideal limit or goal which observation, analysis, and formulation approaches, but never reaches except by an equally paradoxical intellectual intuition. The metaphysical statement does, nevertheless, provide a regulative principle which guides the analysis and the formulation of natural processes just as the soul itself is said to preside over those processes. Its acceptance by the scientist would mean that he agrees with himself to follow rational procedure wherever it takes him, holding his accounts open until all its columns are filled in with observed and analysed material. In this sense it demands the salvaging and clarifying of much that does not at any given stage appear amenable to medical treatment.

The disentangling of this material at present might

follow the principles laid down in Galen's *Utility of the Parts*. The troublesome material in medicine at present is parted between the specialists, is first called functional, as opposed to organic, and is then investigated as neurogenic or psychogenic by the corresponding specialist. It is impossible for the empirical medical man to deny its existence, but it is equally impossible for him to extend his scientific knowledge or principles to cover it without endangering the more solid basis from which he as a scientist starts. The principles of Galen's physiology apparently do not suffer confusion from such an extension. The recognition of the existence of the soul, in fact, demands the recognition of all that goes on in the body, and offers the notion of the body as artist as an intermediary regulative principle for the assimilation of questionable data.

It will be recalled that there are three ways in which the notion of art enters into Galenic physiology, and, in fact, into all Aristotelian science. One of these, found in metaphysics or theology and presented in Galen's rhetoric, is the motion of divine creation according to which the body and its parts are combinations of form and matter made by God's artistry. This is a pleasant metaphysical myth pointing out the subject-matter proper to physiology. Another entry of the notion of art is made when the body itself is recognized as an artist continually building and rebuilding itself by shifting its forms. It is under this general insight that the physiologist detects the structure of the hierarchy of forms in any organ as its four causes, material, formal, efficient, and final. By shifting the heuristic scheme it is possible not only to apply the analysis to sub-organic elements, but also to integrate organs into systems, so that there will result a series of explanations and theories of tissue, organs, and systems.   But Galen sees that this series is not enough for a growing science of physiology.   There will be, for instance, a series of material causes, the four elements for tissues, the tissues for the organs, and the organs for the systems.   But this series is discontinuous, chiefly recording leaps in thought from level to level ; likewise with the other causes.   Galen therefore proposes to introduce a fifth kind of cause, a cause or set of causes to be sought when for any given problem the four causes have been determined.   Causes of the fifth kind may be looked on as the results of the action of the four causes ; as Galen puts it, they are causes " according to what is done or made ".   From this point of view they might be called secondary final causes to distinguish them from the single product which is called the final cause proper. The four causes are found and formulated in the context of a vast and complicated hierarchy of forms and matters, and they are immediate abstractions from this context ;   the fifth causes will then be derivative forms that lie outside the set of primary determinations, accidental forms, if you will.

Galen is here re-introducing the older Greek notion of art in a third way, in which product and artist are external to each other ;   in this way the parts of the body are artists with respect to what they do or make outside themselves.   We may say that the parts of the body are on the one hand intrinsic artists when they make themselves and carry on their own processes, but that they are extrinsic artists also in what they do or make outside themselves ; we may similarly distinguish between the intrinsic and extrinsic arts that they practice. These extrinsic arts with their specific ends or final causes will then be specifications of the general vague notion of the utility of the parts of the body. For any given organ there will be as many arts as there are kinds of operation of that organ on other organs. Further, there will be what might be called co-operative arts in which several organs operate together on each other and on still other organs. These co-operative arts will depend on systems of parts which will be quasi-independent agents in their co-operations. There will be levels and systems of functions which might be called units of bodily economy.

There are certain sciences which have always concerned themselves with this sort of utility, particularly those most closely related to the so-called humanistic studies, where men are the parts and what they do individually and collectively is of primary interest. Political science, political economy, and economics have always been utilitarian in this sense, but they always tend, as Marx has shown, to become thin and insignificant when they lose the specific distinctions and inter-relations between the arts. Generalization without commensurate specification is the besetting temptation. So it has been in the biological sciences whenever the notion of utility in this sense has been applied, as in vitalism. That is the reason that Galen insists that the fifth causes can be investigated only after the four causes have been determined. This order also has another importance. The fifth causes actually come in between the levels of analysis by the

four causes; they do pioneer analytic work in the
interstices between islands of intelligibility already
formulated.   When the fifth causes are thoroughly known
they make a system which can then be translated into
the orthodox fourfold causal scheme.   They are therefore
causes in a dialectical procedure whose aim is the refinement of any Aristotelian formulation.

Recently a great deal of such investigation has been
done in physiology in this country by workers who have
been inspired by L. J. Henderson and J. B. Cannon, and
the new sciences of biophysics and biochemistry have
taken over many of the parts in the programme.   Cannon's
Wisdom of the Body and the monographs upon which it is
based would fit beautifully into Galen's *Utility of Parts*.
Galen's own descriptions of utilities are quaint and so
obvious in some cases that they seem almost incompetent,
until we realize that they are for us simple elementary
illustrative findings of the method.   He wrote a treatise
on the movement of muscles, a strictly physiological
account.   In the *Utility of Parts* he goes on to show
what the various muscles do.   Strictly speaking we may
say that the function of the muscles is to contract, and the
four causes of contraction would give the relevant
physiology of the muscles.   Galen assumes this and then
describes the inter-related operations of, say, the muscles
of the hand to show how it is that the hand is a prehensile
organ capable of grasping, holding, and manipulating
things of all sorts of shapes and sizes.   We still have
vestiges of his descriptions in our anatomical names for
certain muscles, abductor, adductor, buccinator, dilatator,
tensor, extensor, flexor, levator, obturator, pronator,

supinator, rotator. Similarly the stomach functions intrin-sically when it attracts and assimilates nutriment from the blood, but it also secretes juices and digests food for the rest of the body. The endocrine glands have a meta-bolism, but in modern physiology they also secrete and send out hormones. Galen's favourite kind of example is illustrated in his remarks about the lungs ; they carry on respiration and also act as cushions for the heart.

One can see in this the method by which tissues are understood as parts of organs, and organs as parts of systems, and the suggestion is that finally a collection of systems may thus be built into organisms as wholes. The fifth causes come in as approaches to what would now be called the theoretical problem of organization, where modern physiology is admittedly weak. The line of investigation must follow Galen's principles, at least implicitly as it does at present, so that the arts of the digestive system, the nervous system, the circulatory system, the endocrine system, etc., may be articulated and resolved under the final cause of the body as a whole.

But the art principle can be carried still farther into still more troublesome branches of medical science. The body is a whole, but it, like any organ, is also a part entering into processes that carry the arts of life beyond the individual into the natural and the social environment, and for a humanist into the cultural environment. Aristotle had called the rational soul the first entelechy or final cause of the body. The notions of the fifth causes and of the human arts can be combined and found exemplified in geographical medicine, social medicine, industrial medicine, and even legal and religious medicine,

or what the Germans would call a Geisteswissenschaft-
liche Medizin.

The arts were once the vital concern of a circle of
academic sciences, and it was the duty of the scientist to
raise them from the level of mere experience and rule of
thumb to the level of rational intelligibility. The
medieval university was built as a working structure of
faculties, each performing its particular operations upon
the whole field of human arts. It was understood as an
organism with parts and functions like the parts and
functions of the body, and the arts were to be concocted
and sublimated until they were understood and made
capable of being passed on and continued for their true
ends. The transforming and clarifying functions were
nicely distributed between the faculties. The faculty of
the liberal arts distinguished the intellectual from the
useful within the arts by a subtle machinery which dealt
mainly with the symbolically elaborated materials
presented by the arts. The result was, as I have shown
earlier, the construction of propositions and formulae,
and these were then passed on to the three higher faculties
of medicine, law, and theology, where they were organized
in sciences, bodies of theory with known metaphysical
foundations. I have so far been concerned only with the
liberal arts and medicine, but the full story would include
an account of the part that law and theology would play
in contributing to the philosophizing of medicine. These
would have a bearing upon the branches of medicine that
are at present attempting to deal with what might be called
the arts and sciences of the body as a whole. A certain
view of the medieval circle of sciences and arts would

show that many of these modern problems, for instance, in psychiatry, would be relegated to the attention of the faculties of law and theology, and that medicine would select only certain of them for its special attention.   It would follow from this view that with the modern decay of theology as a science and the ever present dangers of the prostitution and degradation of law, the burden falls heavily on medicine, the only faculty that still flourishes. One should view such a situation with alarm, since it represents the overloading of a profession with problems that do not properly belong to it.   This view and alarm are fairly prevalent at present.

I believe the view is romantic and alarmist.   Medicine was in the middle ages as it is now a way of viewing all the arts and their problems.   It was, and is, a universal science, humanistic in its practical aims, but viewing all things through an adequately founded and articulated body of rational doctrine, and confident that it can find solutions to all problems in its own terms.   Its present plight is nothing radically new, though the form in which the problems occur is historically dated and unique as all human and scientific problems are.   The problems of natural adaptation, industry, society, politics, and religion have a medical dimension and should be approached without evasion or contempt by the doctor, who, according to Galen, should also be a philosopher.   The family physician has always had to face a total situation and the profession as a whole may well follow his example.   The present dysfunctioning of theology and law does not raise new problems for medicine in a radical sense ; on the other hand, it renders all medical problems more acute, as the present controversy concerning socialized medicine seems to indicate.

Whatever be the judgment on the professional policies at present there can be little objection, except possibly from the laboratory technician, to the revival of humanism in medicine. There is considerable to be said for the historical thesis that Renaissance humanism as a total cultural pattern grew out of the rapid growth and expansion of the medical faculties in the universities and the consequent naturalization of all learning, but there is more to be said for a counterpart at present which would bring all learning to bear on medicine. This would amount to the reduction of all the sciences to their corresponding arts and would make possible the analysis of modern life, individual, social, and cultural into a system of mutually implicated arts and disciplines. A further small scale analysis of these constituent arts would disclose the values, ends, or final causes, which actuate these arts and the causes that enter into their practice and production. The anthropologist who has been studying primitive cultures and peoples has been disciplining himself in some such objective methods and may be able to transfer some of the theory and technique to our own culture and to our medicine.

If this were done, we should have a basis for discovering not only the first entelechy of the human body, that is the rational soul which presides over all the arts, but we would also have a system of fifth causes which in their turn would become second, third, and fourth entelechies of man, the final causes of man's myriad activities. In such an analysis many forgotten or slurred points in physiology would come to light and be amenable to treatment both scientific and therapeutic.   All this in its present state of chaos and wonder has been loaded into the slender theoretical constructions of the psycho-pathologist and psychiatrist.   Freud working on the therapeutic side of the problem has been rediscovering the liberal arts and making nosograms from the signatures that appear in hysteria.   It is not yet possible to detect the physiological principles that lie in his own scientific subconscious mind.   In the science of psychobiology, as it has developed with Doctor Adolf Meyer and his students, there is even a terminological continuity with the Galenic studies of physiological utilitarianism.   Doctor Meyer would analyse physiological utilities in terms of " ergasias ", workings, doings, or makings that show the hierarchies of form and matter, cause, purpose, and process that mark the arts and their ordering.   Aristotle and Galen exist just under the surface in Doctor Meyer's descriptive accounts of individual cases and a thorough-going formal account of the science waits only on the translation of the former to the latter and the assimilation of the modern findings to the ancient principles.   Doctor Meyer, with many others in this field, leans towards the modern metaphysics of emergent evolution and the pragmatic elaboration of observation.   It is too bad that these popular philosophies are not better understood as disguised and truncated Aristotelianisms.   The sciences that grow precariously out of them fail at crucial points and frustrate their own rational developments.

Perhaps this is the place to generalize all the criticisms of modern medical science that I have made in the course of reviewing the traditional doctrines.   The generalization is simply this : all current science appears to the historian of philosophy and medicine as, on the one hand, a marvellously elaborate accumulation of empirical findings in which the virtue of theoretical simplicity has become a vice, and a most serious obstacle to even the immediate advance of empirical investigation.   Modern empirical science is frustrated science, and its present dogmatic aversion to metaphysics is but a sign of an internal blindness that threatens the value of basic routine research and practice.   I have emphasized the rational and the teleological aspect of Galen's medical theory, not merely because that is Galen's main emphasis, but because he becomes most crucially important for us when he speaks on these matters.   We have learned his curiosity and accuracy in empirical investigations well enough so that we can criticize and correct him there, but we have mistakenly supposed we therefore had the right and duty to ignore him in other matters.   I should like to be equally emphatic on the wholeness of his doctrine.

It is a simple fact, but almost universally ignored in modern thought, that when one loses sight of the end of one's thought and action, the thought and action waver between fanaticism and futility.   The good in itself which confers good on all the means that lead to it, if it is destroyed or ignored, destroys or obscures the goods of the means.   There are analogous principles in all aspects of life and thought.   If one loses the insight which lies at the basis of a science the truths and certainties of that science are no longer attainable either by labour or thought.   The highest activities are said to depend on lower activities, but it is even more true that the lowest activities become diseased and feeble if the higher activities are stopped or hindered.

These statements mean that if the final causes are not known, the lowest correlations will be meaningless. If the rational sciences are neglected the empirical sciences will become black arts and their practices will be quackish. If the speculative, imaginative, and useful arts are confused, then the physiological functions will be disordered.

If medicine is the science of the soul, it is enlightening to recognize that rational science is itself the most important medicine of the soul, a medicine for medicine.

CHAPTER VII

In the preceding chapters I have been following a meta-physical pattern, and it is just, if not merciful, to the reader to give some account of the major themes in it. It may help to place the main thesis of this book in a single perspective without which I fear the exposition will seem hopelessly fragmentary and even more incompetent than it really is. Even this delayed admission may help since it indicates that the main theme has been metaphysical.

Metaphysics is a versatile science. When it is success-ful, it makes fundamental intellectual intuitions available, and in that role it is the handmaid of mysticism. Its propositions are never quite free from the atmosphere of mystery, for the simple reason that their terms, being ultimate, cannot be adequately defined. It is a dialec-tical science, since it provides routes of communication between the relatively ultimate terms of all the other sciences, and it establishes these routes by rational procedures. It is a regulative science because it places the other sciences and also the arts on whatever solid intellectual basis they may potentially have, and it therefore has the right to distribute problems and principles among the sciences according to the best insights of human wisdom that can be made available for any stage of rational discourse.

Metaphysical systems are, on the other hand, merely the repositories of propositions that have at some time in the past recorded and concluded dialectical attempts to make human wisdom effective in the sciences. With their help it is possible, therefore, to recall and revive the insights that have been made available in the past, and it is important to do so if we are to understand any present state of the arts and sciences. The liberal arts, Greek science, and particularly the science and metaphysics of Aristotle and Galen, are heavily loaded with insights, in fact so heavily loaded that the modern intelligence and imagination are pushed to the limits of their capacities in trying to comprehend and exploit the wisdom that lies at the basis of such a tradition as that represented by the medical profession. It is only the petty gesture of a cavalier that relegates this ancient wisdom to the culture museum and decides to face contemporary problems of medicine with naked intelligence. Aristotle and Galen are the mediums through which we see, often unawares, not only our scientific problems of the present, but even the problems of common sense that any practicer of the medical arts has to face daily. Metaphysics is inescapably present in all concrete and practical affairs, and the choice to ignore it can only be the choice to see things darkly. To study Aristotle and Galen is to shine the glass of medicine.

The terms of metaphysics are called transcendental predicates, or more briefly, transcendentals. They are terms that are predicated of all things, if not always explicitly, nevertheless implicitly and necessarily. Their implicit universality explains, on one hand, their apparent emptiness, and on the other, the confusions that follow their neglect. Three are usually recognized in any discourse, true, one, and good. Six were systematically treated in the middle ages, Ens, Unum, Bonum, Verum, Res, and Aliquid. Plato deals with four, Being, One, Same, and Motion. Their number is apparently indefinite, their explicit uses depending on the needs and knowledge of the special occasion ; this variable utility apparently accounts for the differences in the lists at the various times.

They have peculiar properties. First they are predicated of everything, singly and collectively. Second, they are predicated of each other. Third, each is predicated of itself reflexively. Fourth, each is predicated of its opposite. Again traditions and occasions vary in the selection of the properties to be considered, and in the degree of subtlety that will be tolerated in their combinations. Breadth and depth of comprehension actually determine these selections and tolerances.

In my work with the transcendentals I have chosen a middle ground for the present. I recognize the six of the medieval tradition and confine myself to the combinations and propositions that go with the properties that I have named. On this basis there are one hundred distinct possible transcendental propositions, and these can be divided into five groups. Each group includes the propositions that result when one transcendental is taken as subject and all the others are predicated of it. I call this process transcendental conjugation and the resulting groups Verses. With Ens as subject we have the Entiverse, with Unum the Universe, with Bonum the Boniverse, with Verum the Veriverse, and since Res and Aliquid appear to be opposites of one another, the fifth Verse is the Re-ali-verse. This is the limit of elaboration for my capacities in the current conditions under which the intellectual arts are practised. In spite of still remaining dark spots and crowded areas, these verses serve somewhat the function that constellations do for the astronomer. It is possible to observe, place, and describe the planetary motions of the sciences and arts with some degree of precision and a modicum of wisdom.

It is with this system of reference that I have been viewing the medical arts and sciences in the preceding pages. The liberal arts and sciences are concerned with signs and symbols and the levels of generality and abstraction that appear in human thought when symbols are used. They operate, therefore, in the Realiverse where universals (res) are distinguished from particulars (aliquid). The sameness and differences of things appear in this verse as the properties upon which all rational discourse depends. Therefore, the first part of this book, which sets up the liberal arts and applies them to empirical science and the medical arts, gets its fundamental insights from the metaphysical sky through the zodiacal sign called the Realiverse. It is very important that this sign be honoured wholeheartedly if the necessary degrees of detachment in observation and the proper distinctions in therapy are to be preserved. It is only by a thorough education in the liberal arts that the quackeries and literal-minded stupidities in theory and practice can be raised with the subject-matter to the rational level where medicine may be called scientific and professional. The first and perhaps the only essentially important thing that can be done to improve or even to preserve medicine at present is the thorough reconstruction of programmes of liberal education and the first certain proposition that can be laid down as foundation of such a programme is that a liberal education consists in learning the theory and practice of the liberal arts.

I have tried in the beginning of the second part of the book to describe the passage of medicine from the Realiverse to the Veriverse. From the metaphysical point of view this has already happened when the question of the truth or the falsity of the diagnostic or prognostic propositions is raised or when the therapeutic rules are tested for effectiveness. Propositions or patterns of symptoms that have been entertained, expanded, revised, and refitted to the case are still sophistical cobwebs until they are recognized as constituent elements in the medical sciences, but that recognition has the reference to the higher levels of truth implicit in it. Physiology, pathology, and anatomy make that recognition explicit and take on their scientific responsibilities as they become explicitly abstract. I have tried to show by a sort of myth how the Greeks came to recognize the truth values in their arts and sciences. Aristotle and Galen represent the high point of Greek medical science, and with all the noisy and blustering attempts to revolt and overthrow the authorities, we are still working out the details of their fundamental insights. Students in the history of science are steadily transforming the record to show that the great original modern discoveries in physiology and anatomy are without exception rediscoveries of ideas and illustrations of principles in the Aristotelian and Galenic works. One has only to read Harvey and Vesalius to suspect the scandalous superficiality of the special pleaders for modernism who argue against rational dogma. If we are scientific, we are Greek. I am not saying that there is nothing new in modern science ; I am saying that we have yet to recognize and realize the science that has made that novelty possible. The transcendental Verum with its attendant metaphysical questions is the detector and sifter of scientific knowledge.

The transcendental Bonum is hedged about completely for moderns by caveats which mark the failures of incompetent theologians and philosophers in their attempts to make unsystematic and fragmentary use of the Boniverse. Bonum is very intimately associated with Verum, and its fragmentary use tends to confuse both Verses. It was for this reason that the early modern imputation of final causes in science caused a violent revolt against all teleology in behalf of single minded devotion to Verum. But the suppressions of Bonum soon crippled the free search for truth in science, and the last two generations of scientists have been as much embarrassed in their truth claims as the preceding generations were embarrassed in their apologies for design in nature. The present generation has rediscovered utility in nature and Bonum has generated the pragmatic and operational view with its merely strategic and *ad hoc* references to truth in verification.

I have tried to point out the possibilities of regeneration

in these lost dimensions of science by recalling the double reference to truth and utility as it occurs in the Greek origins of theory and practice, namely the arts. The crucial technique here is the abstraction of form, the technique that cured Greek thought of its sophistry. The consequent recognition of formal truths restored the possibilities of acquiring and systematizing material and empirical truths. Similarly the isolation and formulation of formal and final causes validated and strengthened the observation, reasoning, and even experimentation that discovered all four causes and built them into the first foundations of our modern sciences. A recent commentator on Aristotle has thrown this story into a very dramatic biographical account of the father of science, who was first a militant disciple of Plato in his critical war on the sophists, then a metaphysician and logician hammering out the basic conceptions for science, and finally an excited and acute observer of all that nature presented.

The morals to be drawn from the Boniverse at present are various. First, it seems that there should be a fuller realization of the depths and breadth of modern techniques especially in their formal structures and their intellectual contents. This would make it possible to derive more science in the older traditional sense from our technologies, and in turn our scientific findings would have a smoother and less destructive translation into their manifold applications. I have pushed the metaphor of the body as an artist beyond the bounds of moderation because of the importance of seeing the incidence of the Greek arts throughout the various levels of medical art and science.

Second, the contemporary uncertainties in the assumption of determinism in science, interesting as they may be dialectically, are fatal to the scientific enterprise if they are allowed to displace traditional principles, however inadequate their present formulations may be. In the light of the Boniverse these uncertainties appear as the nemetic consequences of the tragic blindness that followed the battles of the teleologists in the seventeenth and eighteenth centuries. With the suppression of final causes there came a confusion and disintegration of the intermediate causes, and in the course of the downward dialectic without benefit of first principles all causes have become evanescent, leaving only the indeterminism of matter. The maxim is : No final causes, no determinism. If it were not for the cyclical nature of dialectic, we might say no determinism, no science ; but with the full cycle about to be consummated we may look for the rediscovery and reconstruction of causal theory and the renaissance of all the sciences on a sounder basis of a determinism honestly limited only by our ignorance.

In the Universe there are many unities. Wherever there is an individual, an indivisible, there is a unity ; wherever there is a form there is a unity ; wherever there is a collection there is a unity. But the modern mind is obsessed with one unity in particular: wherever there is a measure there is a unit. This obsession is the greatest glory that the modern mind has achieved, and the fact that mathematics has progressed by the cultivation of an obsession is not to be brought in as invidious evidence. Special intellectualisms have always been due to cultivation of special neuroses. Obsessions are, however, to be correlated with partial biases and viewed with alarm when they seem to set up absolute limitations. At present there is developing a counter neurosis parading in philosophical discourse as the doctrine of holism. Its subjects hope by cultivating their obsession with wholes to correct the distortions of measurement which they assume to be due to a fixation on parts. In physiology we hear a great deal of speculative talk about the organism as a whole, and a great deal about the schools of physiology that cultivate the neurosis that goes with the obsession of integration. All of this is very unphilosophical. What is needed is a metaphysical licence to measure and specialize, and this itself would show the stations and duties of the specialist with regard to the whole.

This is the state of affairs not only within medicine but also wherever science touches human affairs; perhaps the demand for integration is most articulate in the social sciences where analysis has so long meant merely the art of surveying. Education also has taken to the arts of measurement, and educators are now asking for the humanizing of knowledge to fit measured capacities.

In this last point we have an echo of a useful distinction. There is an ancient distinction between what is clear to us and what is intelligible in itself, and the explanatory aphorism that what is most clear to us is least intelligible in itself, and what is most intelligible in itself is least clear to us. Learning starts with the familiar and moves to the intelligible taking us as far as may be possible with our capacities. The farther we go, the better disciplined we become. The problem of the humanization of knowledge, as it is called, is solved by the human acceptance of the relevant disciplines.

The disciplines relevant to the present mathematical complex and its counter neurosis, holism, are the disciplines of the liberal arts. Training in the quadrivium, the older mathematical arts and sciences, arithmetic, geometry, music, and astronomy, eventually leads to the metaphysical inquiry into the foundations of mathematics in the transcendental Universe (Unum). Training in the trivium, the older logopoetic arts and sciences, grammar, rhetoric, and logic, leads to the metaphysical inquiry into the foundations of physics. These two sciences are at present badly confused because they are attempting to build on the same foundations, and the building of one is preventing or destroying the building of the other. Physics uses the mathematical arts, but it should recognize their subsidiary roles in the Entiverse where its own foundations really are.

Measurement is at present exclusively associated with number and magnitude, so that it may be said that anything whatever is measured if it is brought into one-to-one correspondence with numbers or magnitudes. As a matter of fact, measurement is a much wider conception and is to be found in many universes of discourse where number and measurement are absent, but it may be advisable to examine this current restricted kind of measurement in order to see the objective nature of the tangle we are in. The first step in the building of a metric system is to select and name a unit. This is an act of selection and arbitrary naming as it seems, and its description under present modes is somewhat circular. A given subject-matter is assumed to be undifferentiated, a kind of prime matter capable of receiving distinction. A numerical fiat is laid down in the material, and that becomes a first measure, the unit. Other more or less random selections are made and tentatively named in the same material, and comparisons are made with the unit. As trial and error proceeds, these comparisons fall into elementary analogies between ratios of the names and ratios of the things named. The analogies are also correspondences between the original ratios which relate the many with the unit. The names dictate an order so that any consequent term can be renamed as a certain ratio of the original unit and understood as the product of the application of the ratio to the unit.

The elementary analogies are thus organized into analogies of higher order which are related to the elementary analogies as wholes to parts. Thus the named parts of the material become a system of things, the things form a collection, and the collection can be counted. We have here a one which has measured a material, a many which is the result of the measurement, and a one again which the many together have made. Obviously the collection can become another unit, the first measure of another more inclusive collection, and this larger collection is again a one or unit. Thus it is that the world can be measured.

But contemplation of this result will bring other possibilities to light. The ratios which hold between the members of a collection can be isolated and translated into operations, and these operations can be applied to merely made-up names, which with sufficient ingenuity can be made to bear in their visual appearance and arrangements the order which the ratios or operations give them. This possibility of merely verbal or nominal elaboration frees the metric system from its origin in the naming of material, and with sufficient artificial material can be expanded indefinitely, or if you like into an infinitely extendible metric system. Any operation repeated often enough on an indeterminate matter leads the human mind to the infinite.

But there is also the possibility of building an alternative or many alternative metric systems, and they may be found to be in correspondence so that one can be translated or correlated with another. Thus arithmetic and geometry seem to have grown up side by side, and then later a geometric arithmetic and an arithmetical geometry resulted from the combination and translation of the two. Further, this translation and correlation opened up the possible generalization of the special metric systems so that more and more materials could be brought under their measuring powers. This generality and independence of the metrics could hardly go unexplored by the Greeks and their intellectual descendants. So it has been explored and a higher order of infinity, the infinity of metric systems each infinite in itself, has continually reappeared in the intellectual sky, and again and again there has been rediscovered in the Universe the possibility of a world of mathematical ideas.

The discovery of the possibility that mathematics may have an ideal subject-matter independent of its original metric subject-matter has throughout the history of thought been the first sign of an intellectual crisis. It was such a crisis that Plato recognized and tried to face ; the Pythagoreans had made the discovery and had explored enough to accept the dilemma that the possibility represents, either numbers are the essences in things or they are independent ideas upon which things depend. There is always a tendency to accept the alternative as a disjunction, and this tendency always intensifies the crisis.   Plato and Aristotle both saw that the issue was metaphysical and that it was a fundamental metaphysical issue upon which the possibility of science depends. Similarly Descartes saw the issue, gave it one of the drastic Pythagorean solutions and founded modern mathematical physics in the proposition that corporeal matter is extension ;   analytic geometry exhibits the essences in nature.   The present crisis in mathematics and the physical sciences is due to the acceptance of the same dilemma, and the theological drift of its discussion is merely the sign of an abortive metaphysical attempt to reduce all Verses to the Universe.

In terms of the quadrivium the discovery of an ideal subject-matter for mathematics is only the shift from first and second impositions as they are found in metrical operations to first and second intentions as they are found at present in the theory of functions, the theory of groups, and in the current controversies about the identities and differences of mathematics and logic.   If the quadrivium is dealing with the one and many of the Universe (Unum), the discovery of ideas in mathematics means the ordering of metrical systems in a hierarchy and the analogizing of this hierarchy with the hierarchies of the other Verses ;   for instance with the hierarchy of

universals and particulars in the Realiverse, the hierarchy
of truths in the Veriverse, the hierarchy of causes in the
Boniverse, and finally the hierarchy of essences in the
Entiverse. My diagnosis of these mathematically
generated crises in the history of thought is that mathematical operations and their corresponding insights have
outrun the other sciences and reached a level of development which in mathematics corresponds to the overflow
of intellectual light that we have in the rhetoric of
Plato's Dialogues, the allegorizing of the early middle
ages, and the literary outburst of Elizabethan England.
These overflows originated in non-mathematical Verses
and fell in cascades of analogies on all the fields of science.
The first result was confusion, but the consequences in
many cases and in the course of time were solid advances
in these sciences.   These latter consequences depend to
a considerable extent upon the receptivity of special
sciences to this kind of illumination, and this receptivity
in turn depends upon the formal elaborations and insights
already achieved in their respective fields.

Mathematics has for some time been the overflowing
fountain-head from which our sciences have been receiving their light, and they have reached a considerable
degree of confusion.   The future of our sciences, if I am
correct, depends upon the degree of formal elaboration
that can be quickly achieved within them.   Mathematics
deals with things as one's and many's, and extends itself
to other fields in the application of numbers, points, and
x's, y's, and z's. Even when it escapes immediate
references to these notations and roams free in the
English or Greek alphabet, it still deals with things as if

they were arrays of atoms or units. There are one-many's and many-one's in the Universe that can analogically represent anything in any other Verse. Anything whatever can be thus dealt with in extension. But even on a commonsense level the question can always be asked One what ? and Many what ? and the only answer that comes from the Universe is One-many and Many-one. All other attempted answers are analogical and equivocal reductions. Hence the mathematician's defence of pure mathematics against its adulterations by application.

But there is always one proposition common to any two Verses, and therefore a metaphysical route by which we can pass from one Verse to another. If we allow the inclusion of transcendental opposites, there will be two such propositions. For instance in the Universe, there are the propositions, Unum est Ens and Multa est Ens, and it is by this route that intellectual light can pass without confusion to the other Verses. Since the trans-cendental predicates are mutually predicable, the con-verses of these propositions also exist, Ens est Unum and Ens est Multa, and these propositions strictly belong to the Entiverse. Hidden in these oracular statements there is the suggested solution for the problems of our contem-porary scientific confusion.

The suggestion is that the formal structures within the other Verses be explored and elaborated metaphysically and logically for the reception of mathematical illumina-tion. As Aristotle says, the simple units are not only simples ; they are also natures, and should therefore be analysed and treated under their proper categories. We must return to the questions concerning measurement to see what this means concretely.

The conventional story of the origin of mathematics in the arts of mensuration seems to start with an arbitrary selection of a standard, or " first unit " in a given kind of thing. As a matter of fact, the selection is not wholly arbitrary nor is the kind merely given. A great deal more is known than these blind terms confess. In the first place the kind is actually the determination of either the *a priori* or the preceding in perception or in analysis. In Aristotelian terms a kind is a species of a genus which belongs to a hierarchy of genera and species. The kind to be measured in the limiting case, that is, in a kind that has not been previously measured, is a species whose members have no basis of differentiation except in number. In such a case measurement is a kind of pioneer operation on the unknown, but the base of the operation is very well known in the infimae species and its genus. When the operations are attempted without this base, the result is numerology.

Likewise the selection of the first unit is a technical selection of a material, the artistic selection of a medium which can be informed by the set of ratios into which it must fit when it has received its mathematical form. The magic of counting, weighing, and calibrating, by which matter is transformed into units and measures, is due to the meeting of two Verses, one of which is always the Universe (Unum), and the other of which may be the Entiverse, or one of its modes, say the logic of genus and species as I have shown above. The success of measurement and the combinations of measurement that we call calculation is due to the thoroughly parallel structures of these two Verses and their proportional distributions in the natural world. Measurements are elementary material analogies that ideally belong to the metaphysical analogies that hold between the Verses.

Mathematics when it reaches this analogical musical stage of development will therefore challenge the analogical and formal capacities of the other orders, and it issues such a challenge by threatening the reduction of the other orders to its own one-many terminology. Our own scientific occasion evidences this challenge and threat whenever it is described by the aphorism that all sciences tend to become mathematical. Whenever this is true as in contemporary physics, the failure to control the reduction is due to some failure in the prior analysis of things preparatory to measurement ; it is due to the backwardness of the non-mathematical sciences relative to a special mathematical advance. Such historical misfortunes cry aloud for metaphysical attention.

The point is well illustrated in our present usage with regard to the term, measurement. Mathematics is popularly identified with measurement and calculation, and measurement even in the academic world is dogmatically assumed to be exclusively mathematical. The stricture here is narrowed even farther in technical mathematical practice where any mathematical system is tested by its reduction to number theory. Traditionally measurement is used to cover the application of any rational forms to any material, and the term, ratio, is understood to apply to any rational form, or any reason, as well as the particular relations found only in arithmetic. In the light of the European tradition the challenge of the present mathematical renaissance is a challenge to raise other subject-matters to the level of rational procedure so that their meeting with mathematical procedures whenever measurement occurs will be at least an even battle and ideally a rational integration mirroring in microcosm the interpenetration of the transcendental Verses in macrocosm. It is not metaphysical nonsense to say that mathematics itself is at present in need of measurement by other rational procedures, or that it is in danger of occultation if this is not attempted. The danger here is real and vital. We may have passed the dangers of technocratic ballyhooing, but we have not yet passed the dangers of technocratic theory and practice in higher learning.

I wish it clearly understood that I am not pleading for a return to the middle ages or even to the Greeks in the sense that mathematics should be eliminated or even slowed down in its progress. However, I do think that a new distribution of scholarly energy is indicated. Such a programme would envisage the cultivation of the non-mathematical calculuses, so that more fields of scientific interest could be opened safely for mathematical ordering, and those fields that are now under siege might be strengthened to meet the attack with more intelligence and wisdom. It might seem that the more thorough and vigorous the mathematical attack, the quicker the discovery of rational forms in these fields would be. That is just possible, but only if the mathematician himself becomes metaphysician and is sensitized to other than mathematical order. Without metaphysics the mathematical conquest leads to a romantic and speculative imperialism that withers all that it touches.

The philosophical guild has recently become thoroughly sensitized to the mathematical leadership in science, and to the crises in science that have metaphysical import, but they have not yet found either the mathematical nor the metaphysical method by which the crises can be met. Idealism as a doctrine has disappeared with its occasioning cause, political and economic liberalism. Idealism had the potentialities of a profound humanism which have been only superficially realized in pragmatism, but it was not equal to the scientific and technical problems it had to face. Realism in the modern sense has taken the place of idealism in academic instruction, but its methods are fitted only for microscopic problems in science. Logical positivism starting with the new mathematical logic and now collapsed into the grammar of operations is now having its presumably short career in the sun. These are the contemporary Quixotisms to meet the increasingly recognized metaphysical problems in science. The winds of scientific doctrine still move the metaphysical windmills, and now and then carry away a gallant knight.

By a series of accidents, some of them mathematical, medicine has come to my attention as the medium and perhaps the focus in which the problems of wisdom and science meet. Two years of fairly continuous study have confirmed the first impression that something of importance in philosophy can be done in this medium. It is more doubtful if anything equally important can be done for medicine immediately. Medicine presents an imposing body of knowledge to be acquired, and draws heavily on both the natural sciences and older disciplines for one who is non-professionally interested. It is, therefore, a difficult medium in which to work.

On the other hand, it has retained more of the non-mathematical intelligibilities than any other contemporary body of knowledge. Mathematics through its applications in the laboratory is making its imperialistic attack, but it has by no means conquered yet. Its benefits are felt in the increased willingness of the researchers to think as well as experiment. The present social, economic, and political problems of the profession have served to open up approaches to theoretical problems that have seldom come within the range of the scholar's patient interest. This opening is called the problem of making medical knowledge more available for the use of human-beings, and it has many philosophical dimensions.

This book has been written for a rhetorical purpose, namely to persuade both philosophers and medical men that there are solid matters of great interest and importance for their consideration. It should not end without some statement of a possible programme of study. The main point in the programme is based on the conviction that not only should physicians be philosophers as Galen has it, but philosophers should in due proportion be physicians. In the present state of the intellectual arts, it is difficult to be sure of the definite practical bearing of this opinion. I state the following as my conclusion from exploration in both philosophy and medicine, the former for a considerable time, the latter for the short space of two years. It is chiefly drawn from the considerations in the preceding pages of the present chapter.

Medicine has been a body of knowledge with varying degrees of scientific clarity from the most ancient times. It has in this time built a very imposing tradition with more than the usual concentration of wisdom in it. Throughout the major portion of this time it was dominated by two men, one a philosopher and one a physician. It is not very likely that there is a more rich or important source for the recovery of lost insights than in the writings of these men. On the other hand, there is a striking modern development which somehow grew out of this tradition and in its separate modern career has considerably revised the tradition. This is the development that we are in at present, modern natural science. It is a young development and its contributions to medicine have not had anything like the beneficent effects that they presumably should have. This is partly due to the deadening effects of the tradition itself upon the new techniques and its check upon their acceptance by the profession. One might hope to smash the tradition and allow the full play of the laboratory. That is a well known modern liberal custom, and it has not had in other cases the beneficent effects that might be expected from it. I choose another possibility, namely to recover the doctrines of the tradition in the hope that they can be rendered intelligible enough to absorb modern science within the borders of their ancient wisdom.

This is the reason that I have talked about Aristotle and Galen, and that I now commend them to the attention of others. The suggested next steps follow.

The steps fall on two roads. The first road is the road to the rebuilding of the non-mathematical structures of the natural sciences, those parts of natural science that since the time of Galileo have been relegated to the uncertainties of observation and called subjective. These are not merely the so-called secondary qualities. They include many matters of common sense that still function unrecognized in laboratory procedure, such as the place of instruments in the measuring arts, the assumption of causes, the functions of symbols, the syllogistic processes of reasoning, the order of truths higher than probability, and the ends of the arts within which science is applied. This amounts to the setting up of calculuses of measurement, at least five in number that are different from and necessary to the proper use of mathematics.

This step cannot be taken, except by a genius, without a thorough knowledge of Aristotelian logic, metaphysics, and physics. One can measure our ignorance of these matters by trying to read the *Organon*, the *Metaphysics*, and the *Physics* with sympathy rather than the doctrinaire's contempt. Central to this enterprise is the understanding of the categories, the predicables, the three substances, the four causes, and the six kinds of change. But there is no hope of understanding these without the working familiarity with the logical works, particularly the *Posterior Analytics*, where the nature of a science and the methods by which sciences are constructed is discussed. It is safe to say that nine-tenths of the scientific tradition is a closed book for a modern without a high degree of intellectual assimilation with the mind of its father.

The second road is even more difficult. It is the rationalizing of modern science as it actually goes on, and has gone on, for the last three hundred years. A great deal of this would be impossible without the history that comes before that time, and the intelligibility of this in turn depends upon the Aristotelian terminology and logic. But there is a further aid as far as medicine is concerned in the scientific writings of Galen who bridged for the ancient world the gap between empirical and rational aspects of the natural sciences. There will be found a model which will need revision, but is capable of such revision in manifold ways, so that many modern novelties will seem, as I have said before, to be illustrations rather than refutations of ancient doctrine.

Historically Galen comes at the end of Greek medicine. During its preceding course it had passed through practical, empirical, and speculative phases and stages. The Greek mind had here, as elsewhere, explored most of the possibilities that have appeared and reappeared for the European mind since then. Throughout the period there had been medical sects whose special flairs and flights Galen discusses at length. The latter part of the period had seen the rise of constructive and controlled experiment as well as sharp clinical observation. Medicine was contributing to science in general, and the sciences had made particular and far-reaching contributions to medicine. But in spite of Greek liveliness in the mind, or perhaps on account of it, medicine had fallen into the vices of scholastic specialization. There were schools of medicine in the same sense that there were schools of medicine in this country before the Flexner Reports, places where students could go and study with older practitioners or could read in the scholastic literatures of the sects. They could become specialists, not only in the technical sense where special skill argues special cultivation, but in the theoretical sense where one pseudo-philosophical theory excludes the consideration of another.

Galen brought to medicine a thorough philosophical training and threw all the weight of traditional authority into a critical reformulation of medical science. He used the powerful leverage of the dogmas of Plato and Hippocrates restated and revised to pry loose the petty dogmatisms of the schools. There was almost no corner of medicine that did not undergo his critical organizing process. It was this body of knowledge and principle that became the professional training in the medieval university.

Both roads that I have pointed out for the medical philosopher start with Galen and lead through our modern empiricism and rugged individualism to a new organizing of thought, an organization of thought dogmatic enough to be teachable. In terms of the subject-matter it would mean the establishment of a science of physic in the older sense of the word, a single natural science within whose universal embrace each of the sects and cults of modern experimental and practical science might find its place. The divisions within the science would be of two kinds, those based on the present specialized fields of science, roughly inanimate, animate, and social, and those based on the levels of truths, empirical, practical, rational, formal, and speculative. The former division should be made and systematized by the scientist in the modern sense ; the latter division should be made and organized by the scientist in the ancient sense, or the philosopher in the modern sense.

My notion is that medicine, or physic, would not only be the matrix in which the medical man could trace his signatures and remedies, but also it would turn out to be the philosophy of science that is now being piously and futilely sought for in a thousand universities. As a result research in science on the one hand and metaphysical speculation on the other would be freed from the grotesque burdens which the layman now puts on them. Physic or medicine would recover its lost humanism and its intelligibility *quoad nos* as well as *secundum se*.

There is a modern gnostic cult, anthroposophy, that observes the universe, takes its pulse, diagnoses its troubles, and prescribes its remedies. One of its recent pronouncements is that the year 1930 represents the transference of the responsibilities of the world's affairs from the Archangel Gabriel, who is a kind of celestial politician and sociologist to the Archangel Raphael, who is a kind of cosmic medicine man. The following proposals have no divine authorship that I know of, but they might have been written by the Archangel Raphael's private secretary.

    I. A critical evaluation of the sciences upon which the medical arts depend with special attention to their past uses and their possible future relevance to an integrated science of physic.

    II. The abstraction and reformulation of the first principles in these sciences showing their subordination or interdependence inside a single science.

III. A digest of current working hypotheses, instruments, and techniques in medical research and practice.

IV. A study of measurement in science, numerical and non-numerical.

V. The construction of a rational science and an empirical science of physic based on the preceding studies.

VI. A study of medical casuistry, the applied sciences of medicine, diagnosis, prognosis, therapy.

VII. A study of social medicine, epidemics, preventive medicine, creative medicine, and the proposed agencies for the medical control of society and the social control of medicine.

VIII. A study of the possibilities of a permanent board for the continuous criticism and codification of medical knowledge.

Plato said that society was man writ large ; it may be that some of the large social problems of the present time would appear solved in the study of man who, if Plato is right, must be society writ small.

INDEX

Prediction, 99 ff.
Prognosis, 33, 53, 55 ff., 67 ff., 79, 82, 94 f., 98, 115, 158
Pythagoras, 136, 138

Quadrivium, *v. also* arts, liberal, 6, 20 ff., 26

Rhetoric, *v. also* arts, liberal, 10 ff., 18, 41, 81, 195

"Science," 25 f.
Science of the sciences, 4
Signate matter, 34, 42 f., 51, 79, etc.
Signatures, 32 ff. 49 ff., 102, 122, 157, etc.
Socrates, 23 f.
Soul, the, 164, 169, 172
Speech, figures of, *v. also* rhetoric, 10 ff., 85
Surgery, 60, 77, 83
Sydenham, 89
Symbols, *v. also* signatures, x, 6, 8, 20, 32, 80 ff.
Symptoms, xi, 55 ff.; cc. 3–4, *passim*
Syndrome, 83, 85 ff., 95 ff.

Technology, 44 ff., 52, 103, etc.
Teleology, c. 5, *passim;* 159 ff., 183
Therapeutics, 23, 53, 55 ff., 71, 73 ff., 79, 82, 105 f., 110 f., 115, 158, 179
Transcendentals, 178 ff.
Translation, 9, 11 ff., 27
Trial and error, 29, 84 f., 105, 186
Trivium, *v. also* arts, liberal, 6 ff.

Universals, 17, 62 f.
University, the medieval, 4 ff., 51, 170 f.

Verses, viz. Entiverse, Universe, Boniverse, Veriverse, Realiverse, 179 ff.
Vesalius, 149, 181

Whitehead, A. N., 35, 42, 119

Zeno, 133